"Elliott sheds light on common misconceptions about health and fitness while offering lucid solutions…She outlines a straightforward, understandable—and perhaps most important, *doable*—approach to weight loss that is permanent…Take this book and put it into practice, and you will be transformed for life."

—George Boutros, MD

"Elliot has done the research for us on how to be free to eat and exercise as God intended without all the bondage. Sitting down with this book is like sitting down with your own personal trainer! After reading it, I am inspired and motivated!"

—Denise Glenn,
founder of MotherWise Ministries and
author of *Wisdom for Mothers*

"Everyone should *Kiss Dieting Goodbye* and say *Hello* to this refreshing lifestyle! Change your mind and habits as you follow Elliot's story and directions to living well and losing weight!"

—Mary Lou Retton,
Olympic champion and
mother of four girls

KISS DIETING GOODBYE

Elliott Young

HARVEST HOUSE PUBLISHERS

EUGENE, OREGON

Cover by Left Coast Design, Portland, Oregon

Front and back cover photo © Donald (dk) Kilgore

Advisory

Readers are advised to consult with their physician or other medical practitioner before implementing any suggestion that follows.

This book is not intended to take the place of sound medical advice or to treat specific maladies. Neither the author nor the publisher assumes any liability for possible adverse consequences as a result of the information contained herein.

KISS DIETING GOODBYE
Copyright © 2007 by Elliott Young
Published by Harvest House Publishers
Eugene, Oregon 97402
www.harvesthousepublishers.com

Library of Congress Cataloging-in-Publication Data
Young, Elliott, 1965-
Kiss dieting goodbye / Elliott Young.
    p. cm.
    ISBN-13: 978-0-7369-1895-4 (pbk.)
    ISBN-10: 0-7369-1895-7
    1. Reducing diets—Psychological aspects—Popular works. 2. Weight loss—Psychological aspects—Popular works. 3. Food habits—Psychological aspects—Popular works. I. Title.
    RM222.2.Y677 2007
    613.2'5—dc22
                                                                                                    2006021482

Printed in the United States of America

07 08 09 10 11 12 13 14 15 / VP-CF / 10 9 8 7 6 5 4 3 2 1

To my beloved husband, Ben, with whom I laugh every day.

Acknowledgments

I want to express heartfelt thanks to my amazing editors, Sarah Fuselier and Toni Richmond. Their willingness to make it happen, which sometimes meant kissing some sleep goodbye, was unwavering from start to finish.

Thanks to my precious daughters, who prayed for me every night during the writing of this. I also want to thank Liz Crystal, Amy Hodge, Domenica Catelli, Tara Meyer, Kathrin Milbury, Katherine Purcell, and others unmentioned for their encouragement, prayers, love, and inspiration.

I am so grateful to the incredible staff at Harvest House, especially Terry Glaspey and Carolyn McCready for catching the vision, and Paul Gossard for his insight and attention to detail.

CONTENTS

Foreword
By George Boutros, MD

The quest for beauty and the illusion of control—these two things drive Americans to spend billions every year on fad diet books, online programs, and nutritionless "health" foods. But what they are seeking seems out of reach every time. Why? Because beauty is more than skin-deep—and the illusion of control *is* an illusion.

In my three decades of practicing medicine, I've seen firsthand what the quest for outward perfection can do to health and overall well-being…and it isn't pretty.

Elliott Young has "been there, done that." In *Kiss Dieting Goodbye* she tells her story of falling prey to the illusions of dieting. Through her journey to spiritual, emotional, and physical freedom, Elliott sheds light on common misconceptions about health and fitness while offering lucid solutions. She speaks with authority on why specific popular diets ultimately do not work and outlines a straightforward, understandable—and perhaps most important, *doable*—approach: to weight loss that is permanent, and to having a healthy psychological view of the body and its purposes.

As a friend of Elliott's for many years, I have seen her practice what she preaches. She has proven her own philosophies regarding healthy living, and she inspires others to give the same love and respect to their own bodies.

I am one of those "others," and recently I had the opportunity to see the immeasurable value of this lifestyle approach to well-being played out in my own life. A serious car accident and the discovery of a tumor left my wife and two sons wondering if I'd be okay. I had three surgeries within five days. But within five weeks, I was up and moving again. My doctors were amazed, and they attributed my speedy recovery to the fact that regular exercise, weight training, and nutritious eating habits are an integral part of my life.

That's what *Kiss Dieting Goodbye* is all about—regular people like you and me pursuing health *for life*. Its principles are tried and true, and the science is sound. Take this book and put it into practice, and you will be transformed for life.

And the real beauty of it is, this transformation is so much more than a mere physical one—it's mental, emotional, and spiritual. So get started. You have everything to gain by reading this book and nothing to lose…except excess weight and poor health.

George Boutros, MD
Chief Radiologist, Spring Branch Hospital
Houston, Texas

CHAPTER ONE

KISS FAILURE GOODBYE

With God all things are possible.

In my early 20s, after six months of dating and gradually falling in love with a certain guy, I finally had an awakening. You see, I had been in major denial about a particular area of my life, but now that things were getting serious, I was forced to acknowledge the truth...but not to him, of course. How could I tell my boyfriend that our relationship had not been truly exclusive all those months and that I was torn between two lovers? The fact that I was cheating on him was too much to admit, so I decided to just write him a Dear John letter. Though I was madly in love with this guy, I had been with this other lover much longer. Clearly, this was the easiest and best way to handle the situation.

Only my boyfriend did not take it like a spoonful of stevia. Actually, he did not take it at all. Instead, as soon as he got my letter he drove 90 miles, knocked on my door, sat down opposite me, and told me he loved me unconditionally and whatever the issue was we could work through it together. I finally told him about this third party, sort of hoping he would abandon me for a more deserving and loyal girlfriend. But he was unmoved and insisted we could work it out. I would have to make a choice, to be sure, but if I chose him he would try to help me cut ties.

Ending my love–hate relationship with food was not something that happened overnight, but that day I embarked on a journey of healing that has brought me to a place of freedom today.

Let me to give you a little background on my old lover. In my attempts to shed 15 or 20 pounds in high school—a goal I had formed based on my prepubescent weight—I started counting calories. I was after quick results, of course, so I began cutting back on my intake dramatically. This kind of deprivation was too hard for me to maintain, and I began to cheat...*a lot.* So after a few weeks of feeling like a failure, I resorted to more extreme measures, such as skipping meals and consuming liquids only, which inevitably led to bingeing and then to even more chaos. What resulted was an eating disorder that lasted almost nine years of my life.

This path took its toll on my health, my metabolism, and my self-esteem. Desperation finally forced me to turn to something bigger than myself and what I was going through. By the grace and power of God, I was finally able to let go of temporary solutions, "airbrushed" images, false securities, and the illusion of control. It was an intense spiritual surrender that enabled me to kiss my neurotic eating habits—and the dieting mentality that fostered them—goodbye.

Perhaps only some of you can relate to the extreme practices I was "engaged to," but I would venture to say all of you can relate to a desire to shed unwanted pounds. The two categories are more closely related than you may suspect, as research confirms. Think about it. If the whole idea of "going on a diet" is to help you lose weight (typically as quickly as possible), people who develop eating disorders push dieting to its logical—really, illogical—conclusion. Such people certainly have a skinny leg up on the Atkins, South Beach, and Blood-Type folks. And if we grasp what the dieting mentality ultimately leads to, why aren't we passionately kissing dieting—and the failure and unhealthy habits that come with it—goodbye?

Are You Riding the Diet Roller Coaster?

Even though you are reading this book, some of you are secretly disappointed at the idea of kissing dieting goodbye. The truth is, you've ridden the diet roller coaster for so long you don't know how to get off. You've tasted the exhilaration and have fed on the excitement of starting at the highest height and then plunging to the depths of your scale in a matter of seconds (okay, weeks). It can, indeed, send a surge of power through your whole being.

But here's the problem: You end up right where you started, so you get back in line—stomach still churning from that last ride—only to find that the wait, or weight loss, takes much longer as time goes on. Even so, our culture remains absolutely obsessed with dieting. For some reason beyond reasonable, we'll swallow restrictions, hormonal fluctuation, and often starvation whole—if it means losing weight, even temporarily. We eagerly cut out food groups, eat the same flavorless things day after day, drink unsatisfying diet potions, and pop pills that make our skin crawl in the hopes of quickly losing a few pounds. And yet experience tells us we'll gain them back soon after we quit the unpleasant diet. Why do we do this? Are we just gluttons for punishment?

I suppose it is partly because we enjoy the almost immediate sense of accomplishment that comes with fulfilling a short-term goal—like starting and finishing a book on a plane ride or jogging around the block. This isn't a bad thing in and of itself. But think of the gratification we feel when we set a long-term goal and achieve it. It is far greater in comparison.

Most of us, given the choice, would probably prefer running a mile to running a marathon, but the admiration we hold for someone who has run 26.2 miles without stopping for breakfast or lunch, or to check her voicemail, is undeniable. However, my experience, both personally and as a trainer and weight-loss consultant, tells me that any fairly healthy, somewhat determined person can finish a marathon. (All you have to do to confirm this is simply cheer at the finish line the next time a marathon is staged in your locale. Marathoners come in all different shapes and sizes.)

And let's face it—most worthy accomplishments in life are marathons, not sprints. So this begs the question: Why are we so easily impressed by short-term diet success? Isn't it obvious by now we can lose weight on almost any diet? If we eat only grapefruit or cabbage soup, or go completely carb-free for a few weeks, it is highly likely we will lose weight. But how about something that's actually maintainable and more pleasant? We often act like we're incapable of conceiving a more realistic, livable, and lasting approach when it comes to weight loss. But a lack of ideas isn't really the problem.

Commitment-Phobia

The main problem is one of commitment. Unfortunately, our culture is as commitment-phobic about weight loss as it is about relationships. We may be able to walk down the aisle, but the whole " 'til death do us part" aspect is another story. Around 50 percent of all marriages in this country end in divorce. If I were to pinpoint the biggest contributor to this statistic, it would have to be a lack of commitment. People may say, "We grew apart"…"She's not meeting my needs"…"He's selfish"…and the list goes on. But these are secondary reasons. The same is true in our approach to weight loss.

Americans are losing (and not in the good way) this battle of the bulge because we don't want to go for the long haul. We are all too susceptible to the quick-fix, blab-it-grab-it, get-rich-quick, microwave-it mind-set that has permeated our society. The idea that we can have all we want and have it now *is* incredibly appealing. But as the saying goes, if it's too good to be true, it probably is.

It reminds me of something my youngest said when she was five. "Mommy," she asked, "why would anyone drink *die* Coke?"—referring to Diet Coke, of course. I thought to myself, *What an insightful child!* Okay, so maybe I'm not the most objective person in the world when it comes to my children, but my daughter was definitely onto something. The initial fizz of a Diet Coke feels like the "real thing," but the aftertaste quickly tells us it's not. In the same way, diets promise weight loss and a better derriére, but in reality they only set us up for failure both mentally and physically because of their transient nature. And, unfortunately, when the "die it" is over we tend to really "live it" up because we're sick of the deprivation diets call for.

Extreme deprivation is not possible to maintain in the long run, so the pendulum swings to the other extreme, and we find ourselves indulging in ways we'd never thought of before the diet began. Where has the balance gone in our lives? Many of us are willing to take drugs—regardless of the multiple negative side effects—or even go under the knife before we'll make a commitment to change. These methods are counterintuitive, dangerous, self-sabotaging and, frankly, are not working.

The fact is, as diet programs increase, so does our waistline. We can expect over 76 million Americans to go on a diet this year, but only a scant percentage will keep the weight off. The federally funded Women's Health Initiative reported that women on a diet maintained a mere pound of their weight loss seven years later, and some studies revealed actual weight *gain* in the chronic dieters.[1]

On the whole, the diet and weight-loss industry is leaving millions of us frustrated, dissatisfied, and disillusioned about our health—not to mention the fact that we are spending close to $40 billion a year on dieting and diet-related products with very little to show for it. (By the way, $40 billion yearly is more than the gross national product of most developing countries!)

True Grit

How will we stop the madness? Our one-month or two-month flings with dieting need to be replaced with lifelong commitments to eating sensibly and healthfully. Instead of quick fixes, false promises, pills, and surgery, we need to get highly practical in our approach to weight loss and healthy living. After all, "A little common sense goes a long way." We need to adopt what works! For example, if we have established that the quicker the weight loss, the quicker the regain, maybe we should try the reverse. That doesn't sound too risky, now does it?

Lauren, a woman I worked with a while back, didn't think so. As a personal trainer and weight-loss consultant, I usually start a series of exercise sessions with a goal-setting discussion and questionnaire. Lauren was a weight cycler—someone who loses and regains weight frequently. She told me she was to be in a friend's wedding in several months and, therefore, had hired me to help her lose a large amount of weight in a small amount of time. I simply and emphatically told her, "I don't believe in quick weight loss." She didn't petition or plea-bargain, because this resonated with her common sense. She proceeded to lose one or two pounds a week during the 12 weeks I trained her, and she has kept the weight off for several years now.

You see, committing to change is more "gritty" than dieting. Grit is not just a hip, new buzzword, but a key factor in success. For instance, it's been shown that grit is the premier attribute for surviving the grueling first summer of training at West Point (the "Beast Barracks").[1] It can be defined as the determination to accomplish an ambitious long-term goal despite the inevitable obstacles, or also as persistence in the accomplishment of ends. When someone shows a gritty commitment to exercising and eating well, success is almost assured.[2]

My husband (the boyfriend I was cheating on at the beginning of this story) and I have a "grit" phrase we apply to accomplishing goals and motivating one another to stay on task. We use it in regard to all kinds of priorities, including healthy eating and exercising. The phrase…drumroll, please…is "make it happen." Bridging the gap between knowing that you should do something and actually doing it usually involves overcoming obstacles and having a steady determination. "Make it happen" is a way of saying, "I acknowledge it will not be easy, but I am determined to do it. I'm all about it. I'm gritty."

I admit I'm one of the least "routined" people I know. Our family doesn't ever eat at the same time two nights in a row. (Every now and then I eat dessert before dinner too.) I juggle lots of activities and relationships. I eat out, eat in the car sometimes, and even eat airplane food when I have to. I often exercise at random, unscheduled times of the day. Nonetheless, I've been gritty. I am 15 pounds lighter than on my wedding day 15 years ago, and I lost over 40 pounds of pregnancy weight—twice. I have gained victory over letting food and weight rule my world, and I'm here to testify that you can "make it happen" too. You can be healthy *and* satisfied while getting fit and losing weight.

Does that sound paradoxical right now? I believe it is truly possible to be totally satisfied and simultaneously lose weight. The only hitch is, you must give up the "D" word (diet) and embrace the "C" word (commitment). Let's start by admitting the struggle to God, surrendering our failures, and making a commitment to change our minds, attitudes, and lifestyle.

MAKE IT
happen

1. Ask God to help you embrace a new way of thinking about weight loss.

2. Adopt a "lifer" mentality; throw out "short-term." Your new style is a lifestyle.

3. Take it slow—throw out the quick fix. Remember, a day at a time.

In the style of true grit and your new desire to commit, I give you my favorite minestrone soup recipe. It is labor-intensive and slow, but well worth the wait (sound familiar?). And it's loaded with antioxidants, vitamins, minerals, and phytonutrients. Enjoy!

COMMITESTRONE SOUP
Serves 6-10

1½ quarts cold tap water

1 quart chicken stock (fresh or canned)

1 tablespoon Italian seasoning

¼ cup virgin olive oil

1½ cups (one large) onion, chopped

4-8 garlic cloves, minced

1 cup (2 stalks) celery with leaves, chopped

1½ cups (2 medium) fresh carrots, diced

1 cup (1 medium) fresh zucchini, sliced

1 28-ounce can whole peeled tomatoes

3 teaspoons salt (to your taste)

8 ounces (2 medium) fresh chicken breast halves

½ cup dry red wine (can use cooking wine)

4 ounces (1 medium bunch) fresh spinach, chopped

1 cup Parmesan cheese, freshly grated

1 cup pasta (shells)

2½ cups mixed dry beans

Sort and wash beans thoroughly. Soak beans 4 hours or overnight in water (cover 2 inches above beans). Drain and put in large pot with 1½ quarts cold water, chicken stock, and seasoning. Cover and bring to a boil. Reduce heat to medium low and cook 2 hours.

Ten minutes before beans have completed cooking, heat the olive oil in a large skillet. Sauté the onions, garlic, celery, and carrots until onions are soft (4 minutes). Add sautéd ingredients to cooking beans along with zucchini, tomatoes (chopped with juice), and salt. Cover and cook on low or medium-low heat 1 hour (check at 20 minutes to make sure it isn't boiling strongly).

Add the chicken breasts and dry red wine. Simmer covered 1½ hours. Remove the chicken breasts, discard bones, skin, and fat, and dice the meat. Return to soup. Add the chopped spinach, Parmesan cheese, and pasta. Cook about 8-10 minutes more (test pasta). Remove and refrigerate overnight. Freezes well.

CHAPTER 2

KISS CRAZINESS GOODBYE

The definition of insanity is doing the same thing over and over and expecting different results.

—Albert Einstein

know an adorable husband and wife in their 30s who have stellar children, are committed to church and to their community, pay their taxes on time...you get the picture. The guy is an Ivy Leaguer, and she has a graduate degree in psychology. Smart cats. However, like many good, well-meaning Americans, they have an addiction. No, it is not drugs or alcohol—it is fad diets, or FDs. These are their weapons of mass destruction when it comes to their battles with the bulge.

Apparently, fad diets can be as addictive as adding crack to your morning coffee. No matter how much it costs or how bad they feel afterward, they've gotta see the numbers on their scale take a nosedive just one more time. My FD addict friends got all pumped up about the Body for Life program, which lasted all of three months. Then they were all about the Blood-Type Diet...for a season. They cut out carbs for two months while getting high on protein. This past summer they took a trip to South Beach—and then to the Mediterranean in pursuit of thinness. And off they go again in search of that miraculous diet that will lead them to the Promised Land of permanent weight loss. However, like most Americans they'll be stuck in the Dieting Desert indefinitely. Most FDs sound great on the surface and even seem to work for a little while, but then the bottom falls out. Can you relate to my friends?

Hi-Speed Weight Loss

We can rarely check our e-mail without finding a message about quick weight loss, can we? The mind-set of most dieters is "Get thin quick," and the so-called diet experts are cashing in on this mentality with titles like *The L.A. Shape Diet: The **14-day** Total Weight Loss Plan* or *The **6-day** Body Makeover,* and my favorite: *The **3-Hour** Diet.*

When you plan on losing weight, are you thinking, *Lose 12 pounds in five days?* Or are you more realistic than that, thinking, *I'll lose 12 pounds in 12 days—after all, a pound a day doesn't seem so hard?* Perhaps you don't want to be unduly ambitious. Are you shooting for *five pounds in 12 days at the very least?* If you answered yes to any of these, I want to introduce you to someone.

My girls adore the book *Gullible's Troubles.* It's about Gullible Guineapig, who believes everything he hears. Poor Gullible constantly falls for the outrageous tricks played on him by his Cousin Lila, Aunt Sarah, and Uncle Bernard. For instance, when Aunt Sarah tells him he will become invisible if he eats 50 carrots one after another, he believes her.[1] If you think Gullible's troubles are unique, think again. When it comes to the inflated promises made by the diet gurus of the world, we fall for them hook, line, and sinker.

Beyond our unflappable optimism that diets will work, I'd say one of our main problems is that we're confused; and it's no wonder. Surely you have observed that diet information can be as conflicted as the "no late fee" policy at a certain national video and DVD rental chain:

> *Clerk:* Okay, ma'am, your DVD is due back in two days.
>
> *Me:* But if it's late you won't charge me because there's no late fee, right?
>
> *Clerk:* Well, you have a seven-day grace period after the due date until we start charging you.
>
> *Me:* So my DVD is really due in nine days…and you do have a late fee?
>
> *Clerk:* Actually, we charge you for the purchase of the DVD after nine days.
>
> *(If I had wanted to buy it, why would I pay the rental fee?)*
>
> *Me:* What if I return it after you start charging me for the purchase of the DVD?
>
> *Clerk:* Then, in that case, we charge you a restocking fee of $1.50.
>
> *Me:* So let me get this straight…
>
> *Clerk (grinning):* Good luck.

Confusing, Contradictory, and Can Drive You Crazy

The polarity among the most popular diets is just as mind-blowing, maybe more. One dietist claims carbs are the two-horned culprit of our weight quagmire, and another says eating fruit with meat is a cardinal sin. Atkins promoted eating more protein and not to worry so much about the fat. Pritikin says it's all about eating less fat. D'Adamo warns if your blood type is O, avoid strawberries; if you're type A, avoid tomatoes; type B, avoid avocados; and type AB avoid oranges. (This must be particularly enjoyable when you're shopping and cooking for family or friends.) The insulin-diet pushers don't want us to leave home without the glycemic index. And adding to the barrage of hip diets are the regional diets, which span the globe from the French Women diet to the Asian Women diet and on to the Mediterranean diet—and let's not forget the Sonoma diet. And should we get in the zone, flush our fat, or call Jenny Craig?

Unfortunately, our "scientific" health-related research is equally confusing. We were all scratching our heads after the *New York Times* headlined a 2006 story, "Low-Fat Diet Does Not Cut Health Risks, Study Finds." Other leading newspapers published stories basically touting the same thing: "Fat's not so bad." Apparently, the $415 million federally funded study in question, which tracked 49,000 women from ages 50 to 79 over an eight-year period, showed no reduction in heart disease or cancer risk from eating a low-fat diet. These results seemed to contradict standard medical advice about fat intake.

But just when everyone was about to go on a french-fry-and-milk-shake binge, *Newsweek* did damage control. In an article the very next month, MDs, scientists, and journalists were all backpedaling, dubbing the evidence from the previously mentioned study as altogether inconclusive. They blamed "too much information" as the culprit. Swinging to the other extreme, they practically encouraged us to throw out *any* conclusions from the study.[2]

Well, on some level they're right—we should throw out all-encompassing conclusions. For instance, can we apply the results of the major study with absolute confidence to men, or to persons under 50? No. But on the other hand, we can see from this study that simply reducing *overall* fat intake, which is what these participants did—as opposed to specifically reducing trans and saturated fats—isn't necessarily going to help us out in the long run. (As I will talk about later on, the *kinds* of fats we are eating make all the difference in the world.)

The point is, there are many variables up in the air with health and diet research. And the complexity of these studies can often mask underlying biases as well. We should always bear in mind two questions when we're confronted with health and diet research: Who funded the study? What was their agenda? Unless you're Gullible Guineapig, you know that huge moneymaking industries always have an agenda. Period. I appreciated the candor of Dr. David Freedman, a statistician from the University of California, who said this at the end of the *New York Times* article: "We in the scientific community often give strong advice based on flimsy evidence."[3] In sum, complex research shouldn't wow us when it contradicts conventional wisdom, our common sense, and our experience.

Too Many Choices

We've established that the weight-loss industry is failing us. So what do we do? By no means am I suggesting that we roll over and play dead when it comes to weight loss. It's crystal clear we need to lose weight. What's not crystal clear is what really works. With just a click of the mouse, a plethora of different eating plans is at our fingertips. Our bookstores are filled with rows and rows of diet books. Picking the right approach can be mind-numbing because the number of diets has multiplied exponentially, it seems.

To help sort out the craziness, let's evaluate some of the biggies. The most popular diet methods can be broadly categorized into four main groups—low-carbohydrate/high-protein; low-fat; glycemic-index; and calorie-restriction.

LONGSTANDING CONFUSION

Even when I was a teenager, diets were confusing. Nutrition was not the biggest concern in my family, nor were nutritious foods my preference. I remember grocery shopping for Doritos, Fritos, Chee-tos, Oreos, Spaghet-tiOs, Rolos, and Cheerios. (Maybe that's why nothing in my pantry ends with "os" these days). I used to cherish the day when the Girl Scouts delivered the goods. I was on the cutting edge of Gummi Bears being brought to the U.S. from Germany, and I remember the year when Cookies 'n' Cream became available to the masses. Dinner was often from the Crock-Pot, or it was the Mexican food buffet at the country club.

All of that said, when I needed to lose 10 or 15 pounds in high school, I didn't know where to start. A diet seemed the answer to taming my free-for-all eating. But which diet should I "go on"? It shouldn't be too hard to figure out, right? All the magazines were headlining diets—from the sea-food diet ("I see food, I eat it") to the "If it tastes good, spit it out" diet. The number of diet plans seemed to be utterly overwhelming—and that was 20 years ago.

What About Atkins and the High-Protein Diets?

Atkins and Sugar Busters really gained momentum and peaked in the late '90s, making these low-carb/high-protein diets some of the most popular of our time. South Beach, Somersize (as in Suzanne Somers), and Hamptons fit in here as well. These diets are generally *very* low in carbs and higher in protein and fat. Specifically, in the beginning phase of Atkins, the dieter is limited to 20 grams of carbs per day. (This is ridiculously low.) Then in the maintenance phase, she is allowed 40 to 60 grams of carbs per day (still too low).

These diets continue to attract followers and have affected restaurant cuisine practically everywhere, from the local diner all the way to the upscale sushi restaurant. A popular restaurant in our thriving metropolis even has a whole menu devoted to low-carb choices. Grocery-store aisles are littered with carb-free options as a solution to our growing girth.

I perused the aisles of a standard grocery store and got a good chuckle out of the marketing savvy of these low-carb pushers. A lot of incredibly unhealthy products are selling simply because they are advertised as low-carb. And many product labels boast of low carb counts, putting an actual number on the front. For example, Kraft real mayonnaise boldly advertises on its label that it has a carb count of 0 grams. Kraft fat-free mayonnaise advertises a low count of 2 grams. This trend is a crucial one to investigate. The truth is, when carbs are eliminated or reduced, the product is potentially high in fat—or fat has been added. Processed ingredients are also usually added in to make the product palatable. A good thing to remember when reading labels is that if you take something out you must add something else in, and what's added in is usually worse for us than whatever was taken out. Carbs or no carbs, how can something that is full of hydrogenated fats recommend itself over a handful of carrots?

And one of my favorite discoveries: Many of these low-carb/high-protein diets really aren't for those who exercise a lot. In the introduction to *Sugar Busters,* the authors caution the exercise fanatic and the marathoner, saying, "This diet is probably not for you. High levels of exercise require the foods that generate large quantities of glucose to feed your engine."[4] We haven't even begun to explore the topic of exercise, but I hope you find this statement as amusing as I do. The primary fuel source for exercise is glucose, and this is a glucose-limiting diet. Don't worry—you probably won't have the energy to exercise on this diet anyway. And the book should also have this caution: "If you are planning on thinking, this diet is *probably* not for you," because glucose provides the juice to make our brains function properly as well.

Another beef with these diets is the idea we should steer clear of potatoes, carrots, and beets in order to make more room for steak, lamb chops, and cheese. In reality, protein is supposed to comprise about 10 to 15 percent of our calories. It doesn't matter how much these "experts" like to point to our carnivorous ancestors, God's original provision for us was "every seed-bearing plant on the face of the whole earth and every tree that has fruit with seed in it. They will be yours for food."[5] The plants of the garden were abundant, accessible, and satisfied the energy needs of Adam and Eve and everyone up to the days of Noah. It wasn't until after the flood that God added meat to our diets.[6]

One needs merely to glance at almost any food-guide pyramid—there are a ton of different ones out there nowadays—to observe that carbs comprise a greater part of the recommendations. This is precisely why people who have lost weight on a high-protein diet tend to look unfit and ill. These diets can be toxic to the kidneys and potentially dangerous to the heart.

From Pritikin to Fat Flush

The Pritikin Principle, Dean Ornish's Life Choice Diet, and Fat Flush are popular representatives of the next big category. Low-fat diet proponents typically recommend eliminating as much fat as possible from the foods we eat. And the low-fat and fat-free product influx is not to be overshadowed by its carb-free competitors.

My husband recently came home from a road trip with an empty package of low-fat beef jerky. (It's disturbing what he eats when I'm not around.) "What exactly *is* that made of?" I inquired as I read him the ingredients (as if he wanted to know post-digestion). This is the question we must ask when something that *should* have fat in it is fat-free. For example, fat-free butter, fat-free ice cream, and fat-free cheese are all twisted sisters of their natural counterparts. It may taste *delicioso,* but what exactly is it? Processed, fake stuff that your body will not be thanking you for later.

I ran into a friend at the market the other day, and he was impressed by my cart full of fresh produce and other healthy fare. I assured him that I sometimes buy ice cream too, and as I was reaching for it at the bottom of my cart, he commented, "Yeah, and I'm sure it's fat-free." Producing my carton, I surprised him with a firm "Never!"

Don't get me wrong—too much fat can wreak havoc on our bodies, contributing to weight problems, heart disease—which is our nation's number one killer of men and women—and a host of other problems. Twenty years ago we were eating fat like it was going out of style...and then it actually did. My main issue with these low-fat diets is that they usually don't differentiate between good and bad fats. We should be eating almost no trans and hydrogenated fats, but we need to add the natural, omega-3 fatty acids back into our diets (see chapter 9).

What's Wrong with the Zone and the Glucose Revolution?

Another category that has gained serious momentum in the last several years is the low-glycemic diets, such as the Zone, the New Glucose Revolution, and the Glycemic Index Diet. Their claim is that high-glycemic foods, or carbohydrates that quickly break down during digestion, are a cause of weight gain. The glycemic index assigns a numeric description to a certain food based on the body's blood glucose response to it. While this does have practical applications for diabetics, the whole premise is a bit illogical. If we're truly concerned with health in terms of sugar ingestion, then it stands to reason we would be just as concerned with health in terms of nutrient density (in simple terms, how much nutrition a food contains). This is where the glycemic index quickly breaks down.

For example, green grapes and green peas have a higher glycemic-index (GI) value than peanut M&Ms. Raw cantaloupe has a GI value of 65, and instant vanilla pudding made with a box of powder and some milk has a GI value of 40. (Now, which do you think is healthier?)

Besides these oddities, the latest information relating to this method is showing that the GI values between apples and apples (not apples and oranges) can vary as much as the caffeine content in a tall Starbucks coffee of the day.

Jenny Craig and Her Calorie-Counting Friends

The last group, but the classic approach with no small following, is the calorie-restriction or low-calorie diet. The Weight Watchers program takes on this approach, as does Jenny Craig. These are some of the more logical diets. Physiology 101 asserts that if you take in more than you expend, you will expand. Therefore, calories count. And I do like the fact that Weight Watchers involves group support and accountability. It is also a more savory alternative than Jenny Craig, which limits calories by requiring that you eat prepackaged—that is, expensive and taste-less—foods, not to mention the fact that there is no research supporting Jenny Craig's results. But keeping up with points, as is required in Weight Watchers, necessitates micromanagement—counting and recording your consumption—which is fraught with problems.

Typically, whenever I ask clients to tell me what they have been eating in the last week, they cannot remember. When I request they keep a journal of their food intake over the next couple of days, you would think I was asking them to hop on the scale for a weigh-in (which, by the way, I don't do). It seems to be too personal, too tedious, or too irrelevant. It's like pulling teeth, but I can occasionally extract a day's worth of their food consumption in order to assess if there are any weight-loss-sabotaging patterns. Chances are, though, they will be on especially good behavior that day since it's going "on the record."

Most people haven't the foggiest idea how many calories must be burned up to lose a pound anyway. They would be even less likely to know how many calories, based on their height and weight, they should consume daily to lose a pound a week. And honestly, I'm bored just thinking about it all. Applying mathematical formulas to our eating takes the fun out of it, and food is partly about enjoyment. Just as God designed sex for procreation *and* pleasure, He gave us food for sustenance *and* pleasure. On both counts, there is functionality and enjoyment, and the two are intrinsically intertwined. The human race would not be reproducing if God had not made the method pleasing. Likewise, we should delight in the tastes, textures, aromas, and colors of food, which engage all of our senses. If food and sex were not so pleasurable, the human race might have ended long ago.

But beyond all that, the main reason low-calorie diets rarely work for us long-term has to do with our metabolism. The metabolism has a mind of its own. If you decide to consume 2000 calories a day, your metabolism will then decide to burn 2000 calories a day. It's kind of like gambling. In a more extreme case, if you limit your intake to 1100 calories a day, your metabolism will call your bluff and go into preservation mode—meaning your body will hold on for dear life to that excess fat you're trying to burn. We have to outsmart our metabolism so it will respond favorably by *burning up* the fuel, rather than storing it.

Why Diets Won't Win in the Long Run

Many of you reading this have tried one or more of these diet methods in an effort to lose weight and have found at the end of six months that all you lost was time and money. And what you gained in the aftermath was just more pounds.

Let's review some of the reasons these diets fail us:

- *Low-carb/high-protein diets* fail us because our bodies need carbs in order to burn calories (for fuel). Plus, it goes against all health sense to rely on foods that are often full of saturated fat.

- *Low-fat diets* fail us because we end up consuming more total calories from other sources, especially sugar, in an attempt to satisfy our taste buds. Also, we end up cutting out good, heart-healthy fats along with the bad.

- *Glycemic-index diets* fail us because they sometimes contradict pure common sense: How could peanut M&Ms be better for weight loss than fresh grapes? The GI method is also suspect because of the tremendous variances in food types, as well as the impact of different cooking methods.

- *Low-calorie diets* fail us because we will not last long counting every single calorie, and our metabolism will outsmart us anyway.

All of these diets potentially discourage the eating of some foods that are packed with nutritious vitamins, minerals, antioxidants, and phytonutrients. These vitamins and nutrients are essential if we're going to have healthy, energetic bodies that function and burn fat properly—which, let's face it, is our immediate goal. Lastly, diets put the emphasis on recording, micromanaging, or obsessing over what we put in our mouths, which only leads us to think about food more…as if we weren't thinking about it enough to begin with.

All we have to do is look around to see that the diet industry has not positively impacted our overweight epidemic. On the whole, it's because their main focus is on restriction. Many of us have become fat-phobic, carb-phobic, calorie-phobic, or a combination of the three, when none of these are the enemy. We have established we can gain weight by eating too much of certain things, and the reverse of that would seem to be we can lose weight by eating less of those things. But are we eating less of the wrong foods and eating more of the good ones? No. Are we losing weight and keeping it off? Again, no. And, most importantly, are we improving our health? I think not.

To quote a phrase that has become a Young household favorite, "I am all astonishment!" (These words come from Jane Austen's *Pride and Prejudice*.) This phrase encapsulates how I feel about our obsession with diets. After decades of dieting, educated people are still acting out Einstein's definition of insanity: doing the same thing over and over again and expecting different results. I am all astonishment that the diet game has such appeal, in spite of its underwhelming results. After all the often-cited statistics proving the long-term ineffectiveness of dieting, people are still willing to play diet roulette and risk losing their health, hard-earned money, freedom to choose…and the list goes on! I am also all astonishment that people will enthusiastically buy into the latest diet trend, even though it completely contradicts the recommendations of the last diet they tried. Surely our reasons for persisting in this madness are more than skin deep. In the next chapter we'll dive into the inner workings of what I call *idietry*.

MAKE IT *happen*

Here's How You Can Begin to Kiss Crazy Dieting Goodbye

1. Stop buying into fad diets.

2. Get in touch with your body: hunger, fluctuations, and responses.

3. Set simple, attainable, and reasonable goals, with a short-term goal of about a pound a week most weeks, until you reach your long-term goal weight (see the body-mass index in the Resources section).

4. Recruit support by communicating your goals with the people around you.

ONE-DISH CHICKEN AND VEGGIES

Serves 4

3-4 boneless, skinless chicken breasts, cut lengthwise into strips (about three strips per breast)

8 sun-dried tomatoes in olive oil (cut in half) or ¼ cup julienne sundried tomatoes

2 cups small red potatoes, parboiled (boil in water for about 7 or 8 minutes)

1 cup baby carrots

1 cup broccoli florets

1 cup cauliflower florets

¼ cup chopped onions

5 cloves garlic, peeled and chopped (or 2 ½ teaspoons jarred cut garlic)

3-4 tablespoons fresh chopped rosemary

3-4 tablespoons fresh chopped thyme (optional)

3 tablespoons olive oil

2 tablespoons balsamic vinegar

Preheat oven to 350 degrees. Lightly spray a 9 x 13 baking dish or pan with olive oil. Put sun-dried tomatoes in first. Add chicken breasts. Spread garlic on chicken pieces. Add all other ingredients to dish. Whisk oil and vinegar together and pour over chicken and veggies. Cover and bake 1 hour (uncover for the last 10 minutes). The veggies will be a bit crunchy, which I prefer. If you like them softer, add some water (¼ cup) to the dish before putting it in the oven.

A friend gave me this recipe years ago, and I have modified it to fit my ingredient preferences. My girls love all the veggies in this, but you could use any. I have used green beans cut in half, asparagus, and red bell pepper slices in place of other veggies. You could also experiment with the herbs. It is a fun one to play with.

Carrots and potatoes are good for you, especially when mixed with protein. Carrots are an outstanding source of antioxidants, which help protect against cancer and cardiovascular disease, and they are a good source of fiber. Potatoes are a good source of numerous nutrients, including potassium, vitamins C and B_6, and fiber.

CHAPTER THREE

Kiss Idietry Goodbye

**Forget the former things;
do not dwell on the past.**

I sn't it ironic that our first act of rebellion against God involved food? The Bible tells us that in the beginning "the LORD God made all kinds of trees grow out of the ground—trees that were pleasing to the eye and good for food."[1] Something God created for sustenance and pleasure was quickly corrupted by Eve's craving for more.

The Garden of Eatin'

Today, we are still enticed by the power of the "apple"—the idea of security, comfort, and satisfaction apart from the One who gives us all good things, including food. But shame always seems to follow these fruitless grasps at fulfillment, doesn't it?

We are well aware by now that dieting is not panning out physically. The truth is, dieting has left us emotionally exhausted and spiritually defeated as well. Why? Because we've not only failed ourselves, but we feel we have also let God down with our lack of self-control. So what do we do? If at first we don't succeed, we pick ourselves up and diet again, thinking this time we really will feel better about ourselves; this time we really will be in control; this time we really will succeed. After all, it's only for a little while anyway.

Getting to the root of the issue, I think the three things I just listed are some of the most prominent reasons we "go on diets." Let's look at each of them in greater detail.

1. We Are Desperately Unhappy with Ourselves

One of my clients told me something I will never forget. She said, "I woke up one day, and I was surprised to find I was 50 years old and 50 pounds overweight." We seem to forget so easily that bad habits are established over time and that packing on pounds is not an overnight phenomenon. For one person, seeing his or her image in a photograph is a reality check. And for another, the misguided words, "When are you expecting?" do the trick. Sometimes it takes something more serious, like a divorce or a health scare, to bring us to that "I can't stand this anymore" feeling. But for most of us, the brutal honesty of the scale can send us into a tailspin.

A Rude Awakening

A whole plethora of circumstances can trigger self-evaluation, self-criticism, and self-focus, which aren't all bad, but the sudden feeling of panic reflects our final descent from indifference or denial to self-loathing. Realizing we have a weight problem should provide a wake-up call, not a panic attack. It is this panic mode that ultimately sets us up for the diet mentality. We have been stuffing our emotions and tending to other aspects of our lives—sometimes worthy ones—and paying no mind to the creeping weight gain. Then one day we have a road-to-Damascus, terrible-twos-my-child's-*not*-really-an-angel moment, and we are finally brought to our knees in desperation.

My wake-up call was finally being confronted with the unhealthy pattern I'd established in my relationships with the opposite sex. I was forced to ask myself whether I wanted to spend the rest of my life shutting out, breaking up, making excuses, and living in isolation because of my body image, weight issues, and food dependency. Or did I want to change, receive forgiveness, be vulnerable, and be loved? Eventually, I got desperate enough to surrender my old ways—which had ceased to be fun and fulfilling long before anyway—and change. Would it get me to my goal weight? I wasn't sure at the time, but that was a risk I finally was willing to take. It was a risk that led to my ultimate freedom.

So my question to you is, are you desperate yet? I sure hope so. Desperation is a good thing when we channel it toward change.

2. The Illusion of Control and the Appeal of Autopilot

In spite of the difficulties and dictates of diets, mindless adherence is unbelievably appealing. To tweak a famous C.S. Lewis phrase, *dieting is a tame lion.* In other words, dieting is really the easy way out. It's all roar and no bite. It takes far less discipline to turn on the autopilot and go through the motions of a diet than it does to actually change our ways for good. We do not have to buy wholly and philosophically into a diet because it's a short-term method. And besides, someone else patented it, so there is no personal exploration, conviction, or repentance when it fails.

We know that doing something by rote requires little heart, mind, strength, and soul, yet what's so incredible is that we still feel this deep and inflated sense of personal achievement when we are able to confine our desires and follow a diet for a while. The truth is, it appeals so much to our pride. Notice the middle letter of *pride,* and you'll see what dieting is all about. It is really all about "I."

In a little play on words, I have dubbed this concept *idietry.* We set ourselves up as the god of our stomachs, and diets provide our ultimate Law to follow. And when we are able to abide by the Diet Law, our pride is puffed up all the more. What pleasure we take in dotting the i's when tracking caloric consumption. However, our plans always fall short, and we can see the evidence of this on our thighs! This is because it's impossible to follow our Diet Law perfectly. Isn't it ironic how attracted to rules we are even though we aren't very good at keeping them?

Inevitably, instead of being masters at the Diet Law, we find it ends up mastering us. The control we thought we had was nothing more than an illusion. This is always the way with trying to keep rules, isn't it? Look at our spiritual lives: We can't always do the right thing, because we are flawed human beings. Why would dieting be any different? We have such high expectations for ourselves when we start a new diet, stroking our egos whenever we're behaving. But when the inevitable failure happens and we begin to err, we castigate and despise ourselves. So then what do we do? We tighten the reins with new rules, which only leads to more failure.

When I started dieting in my teens, I never felt successful because I fudged (literally) way too much. With the Diet Law as my ultimate standard, I cratered way more than I cleaved to its rules and regulations. It seemed beyond my ability to be successful. (Is this sounding familiar?) Actually, the apostle Paul addressed this type of thing in his letter to the Romans: "What I don't understand about myself is that I decide one way, but then I act another, doing things I absolutely despise."[2] Paul certainly seemed to have read my mail.

But it doesn't stop there. We don't have to continue living in this cycle. Take a look at this part:

> So, my friends, this is something like what has taken place with you. When Christ died he took that entire rule-dominated way of life down with him and left it in the tomb....For as long as we lived that old way of life...sin was calling most of the shots as the old law code hemmed us in. And this made us all the more rebellious....But now that we're no longer shackled to that domineering mate of sin, and out from under all those oppressive regulations and fine print, we're free to live a new life in the freedom of God.[3]

Did you see that? We have been released from the old way of life. That spells freedom from being confined by the Law, as well as freedom to live *rightly* in this new way of life. There's a huge difference between the two.

So, to apply this to eating, are you trying to follow a strict set of Diet Laws, or are you really free to enjoy *in moderation* the nourishing, satisfying foods God gave us, not so that we can just survive, but so that we can live life to the fullest?

There's Freedom in Boundaries

I married one of the most graceful persons I've ever known. No, I don't mean that my husband does pirouettes around our living room. What I mean is that, hats off to him, he displays acceptance and love to others—especially me—when I do nothing to deserve it (and often when I do things that deserve the very opposite). This stems from his ever-growing understanding that God treats His children with *grace* (which some refer to as divine unmerited favor). My husband knows he can mess up, but God still loves him and wants to give him good things.

In spite of this freedom he knows he has, my guy is also one of the most upright persons I have ever known. He says "Yes," not perfectly, but consistently, to doing the right thing on a daily basis. One fine day he got all excited about implementing a day of rest into our family's week. Being the laid-back wife I am, I immediately jumped on board...No, that's not actually how it happened. I was very hesitant at first. The focus of a day of rest, or a Sabbath, in my mind was about laws. I guess I imagined it as the Pharisees did back in the day.

I had viewed it as just a bunch of restrictions and demands to follow. To me, it was *no* phones, *no* computers, *no* errands, *no* birthday parties, *no* commitments—saying *no, no, no.* To my husband, however, it was all about more freedom—freedom *from* producing, *from* consuming, *from* the technology that seems to rule us more and more every day, *from* creating, *from* "business as usual"...and, more importantly, freedom *from* worry: *from, from, from.* In other words, not bound *to,* but freedom *from.*

Now, on Sabbath afternoons we take a break from the often frantic pace of our weekdays, and we relax. After almost two years of falling into a Sabbath rhythm, the benefits have far outweighed the perceived sacrifices. My mind and body delight in this short but meaningful reprieve. Astonishingly, our children have commented that Sabbath day is their favorite day of the week. They say things like, "I love it when we are at home for the day"; "I love it when we don't have to be somewhere." And these comments are from the same kids who were less than excited, to put it mildly, about the concept originally.

And I'm finally getting it too. There are, to be sure, certain practices we try to abide by, such as turning off phones, TVs, computers, and radios; leaving the dirty dishes and sweaty clothes; and RSVP'ing "no" to stuff on that day. But these rules really are guidelines to promote freedom—and not laws to be followed *or else*.

The essence of that story is similar to the freedom I have experienced since the day I decided to stop dieting. Put simply, I decided diet rules were dumb and change was smart. Maybe we should take heed to something the very wise St. Paul points out in his letter to the Colossians:

> "Don't touch this! Don't taste that! Don't go near this!" Do you think things that are here today and gone tomorrow are worth that kind of attention? Such things sound impressive if said in a deep enough voice. They even give the illusion of being pious and humble and ascetic. But they're just another way of showing off, making yourselves look important.[4]

Are you stuck in a rut of rules where all you hear is, "Don't touch that dressing! Do you know how many calories are in that?" "Don't taste that pasta! That will go straight to your hips!" "Don't go near that chocolate! Yes, you heard me!" It's time to be free, my friend.

3. It's a Short-Term Gig

The last reason we go on diets is because we know that when it's all said and done, we'll get to go back to the pleasure-abusing, all-you-can-eat lifestyle.

In case you hadn't noticed, eating is an important part of living. It's not like alcohol, where if we're temped to overdo it we can work on just avoiding it altogether. Overeaters don't have the option of practicing complete abstinence. We must face our foods. And instead of developing and practicing self-control in our long-term eating habits, we would often rather restrict ourselves for the short-term. And since we're all about the quick fix, let me ask you a question: Why are we not all going out and getting liposuction? After all, what seems easier, liposuctioning your fat out or dieting? Obviously, lipo would be quicker. Let me add another question: What seems easier, dieting for two months or changing for life? Of course, this is where dieting wins out. But the truth is, changing for life is the most logical, most effective, and healthiest way to lose weight and keep it off.

So why are we still dieting? Here's my take from my own experience: We don't want to surrender the perceived control a diet gives us, and we are morbidly afraid of the pain that long-term discipline implies. But someone must lovingly speak the truth, so here goes: There are no quick, easy routes to permanent weight loss. It's a lot like...let's see...life!

What *Does* It Take to Win the Weight-Loss War?

I was at a local coffeehouse recently, enjoying my caffeine-enhanced writing time, when a gentleman (I'll give him the benefit of the doubt) sat down next to me and offered himself as a conversation partner. He opened with this: "I read the other day that happiness is the absence of pain. That's good, isn't it?" To which I countered, "C.S. Lewis says pain is the megaphone through which God speaks." Instead of shutting things down, as I thought it would, this inspired him. He proceeded to tell me he was not too happy with God about pain and suffering. Though I held my tongue, I was thinking of a line from the movie *The Princess Bride*, when dear Wesley tells Princess Buttercup, "Life is pain, Highness, and anyone who says differently is selling something."

I'm not preaching "no pain, no gain," but when it comes to weight loss, I have some good news and some bad news. Let's start with the bad news: Changing is much more painful than dieting. Our bad habits are like old friends, familiar and comfortable. We can go on a trip and leave them behind for a short while, but don't ask us to say goodbye to them forever. Saying goodbye means giving them up for good, and that hurts. It can also be scary because we don't know what the future will really be like without them.

We could draw a parallel to our view of God. Many people give no thought to the possibility of a higher being, or they profess to having an intellectual hang-up that inhibits their truly consenting to God's existence. One popular beef is, "Why would a good God allow bad things like hell and starvation and war?" Or another famous argument is, "Why would there only be one way to heaven?" When the point is pressed, though, the intellectual smokescreen often comes down, and the bottom line is actually about personal suffering and surrender. We don't want a higher authority to whom we have to answer. In that case, we might have to give up sex outside of marriage or cheating on our income taxes or sleeping in or working on the Sabbath; or it might cost us something financially; or we might have to change the way we view our bodies and our eating habits. Yep! The bottom line, if we want to be brutally honest, is this: We want to be our own God, and we want life to be as painless as possible.

The reality is, life is much more painful without God. You can suffer with Him, or you can suffer without Him. No matter what some of the telepreachers are selling, life involves hardship. But the hardships and the sufferings chisel us into beautiful creatures who can boldly face life's tsunamis as well as the daily grind because we've learned to think more like our Creator, who sees the big picture. Take a look at this passage from Scripture:

> Since Jesus went through everything you're going through and more, learn to think like him. Think of your sufferings as a weaning from that old sinful habit of always expecting to get your own way. Then you'll be able to live out your days free to pursue what God wants instead of being tyrannized by what you want.[5]

Losing weight permanently demands more of us than temporary robotic compliance. It requires permanent change, and permanent change in any area of our lives requires conviction, humility, and surrender. But the good news is that it leads to ultimate liberation. And here's some more good news: God will give you the grace you need to change. He is opposed to the proud but gives grace to the humble,[6] and we need grace every day for the fight against gluttony and laziness. We must humble ourselves under the hand of God, ask Him for help, wisdom, and self-control; and here's the kicker, we've got to ask for it every day for the rest of our lives.

It seems contradictory—this idea of freedom in surrender—but it's a tension we must embrace if we truly seek to be free. God is not a tame lion, but He is good, and He has the best in store for those who choose His way of life, which is the best possible way to live.

The Path of Freedom

Weight loss, like life, involves hardship and requires faithfulness. You can continue to buy into the idea that there is a quick and easy way to lose weight—dieting—but after many failed attempts, you might have realized dieting is actually the more frustrating approach. We have to embrace the long-term struggle because, ultimately, we get out of it what we put into it. If you put a short amount of time, little contemplation, and minimal effort toward change, the results are short-lived. Honestly, the high-maintenance, restrictive diets can be much more painful physically, but the approach of lifestyle change, surrender, and walking in self-control can be painful both spiritually and emotionally.

It is a long, arduous path, but it's paved with common sense. There will be some detours and roadblocks along the way, but the path can be obvious and straightforward. Consider, in contrast, the irony of the dieting roller coaster. You have been eating the wrong things and overeating for quite some time (it takes time to gain weight)—and now suddenly you are going to restrict and micromanage everything you put into your mouth. This is like asking you to start exercising for an hour, five to six days a week, from scratch. Most fitness experts don't recommend this approach (and if they do, run, jog, or walk the other way). You would be sore, exhausted, frustrated, and possibly injured. This is why diets and the weight loss that may accompany them are not sustainable or practical. Long-term weight loss includes long-term weight maintenance. And therefore a significant change in thinking and methods must occur.

Health, Joy, and Grace

If your primary goal in losing weight is health, you are on the right track! We should want to lose weight, not only to look better, but in order to enjoy all the days God has given us to the fullest. And enjoying life to the fullest means avoiding the disease and addiction associated with being overweight. With this new way of eating and moving, a weight loss of one to two pounds a week is reasonable and achievable most weeks. Don't be discouraged if you don't lose any weight some weeks. Compared to your former overconsuming and undermoving ways, weight maintenance is a great goal some weeks! Water retention can also be a factor, especially—for my girlfriends reading this—during that time of the month. Our hormones aren't the only thing fluctuating. I gain four to five temporary pounds every single month. I expect it, and I accept it for those few days.

The main thing you must do is get in touch with your body and know its rhythms and responses. Some foods cause salt retention, constipation, or bloating, none of which tip the scale in your favor. Holidays are good days for maintaining instead of losing or gaining. Cut yourself some slack, and then get back on track!

I fully embrace grace-driven weight loss. We need God's grace to help us press on, and we need to have grace with ourselves. I love the verse that says grace trumps judgment![7] We are all going to blow our eating-well goals sometimes, whether it's for a meal, a day, or a week. It's not about perfection—that's a dumb diet. (More about perfection in the next chapter.) And it's not even about perfect adherence to the new way, but rather about our response when—not if—we blow it. Will you throw in the towel at lunch because you blew it at breakfast, or can you get over it and journey onward?

As in our spiritual journey, we will not be able to live perfectly. So just because we can't, should we then throw all attempts to the wind and *party*, as the apostle Paul asks?[8] Of course not—that's a dead end. We have tremendous spiritual and physical problems because we don't know how to receive grace. And by the way, you have to receive it to give it. I have met so many people who are rule-keepers at heart. They see life as just rules to be followed. No wonder they are sullen, joyless, and thankless.

The *good* news I'm presenting here in our approach to weight loss is that we are throwing rule-keeping and restriction down the disposal for good. We get to put aside the calorie counting, the obsession with carb-free/fat-free eating, and the eliminating and dissecting of certain foods. No more beating ourselves up because we don't measure up.

Nor am I going to dole out a plethora of absolutes, such as *never* eating in your car or *always* drinking eight 8-ounce glasses of water every day (though these are both good goals). The truth is, many of us have demanding jobs, demanding friendships, spouses (also demanding from time to time), and children (ditto). Most of us wear multiple hats as corporate men and women, volunteers, mentors, parents, and so on—and just as dieting sets us up for failure, so does inflexibility. I'm a firm believer in absolute truth, but in adopting a new weight-loss approach, I think it is helpful to realize that our "non-negotiables" will vary from person to person. One size does not fit all.

Believe in the Process

In counseling and training people over the past ten years, I have observed some common denominators among those who keep the weight off. I'll be sharing these with you. And instead of laws of micro-management, I have some critical strategies that, when applied, will take the pounds off in a sensible way. I think we deserve a smart, tasteful, and downright enjoyable approach to weight loss, don't you?

That's why we're not going to calculate caloric expenditure based on your weight, activity level, and so on. It's tedious and time-consuming, but more importantly, so small-picture! Do you want to know the easiest way to figure out if you are eating too much or too little? (It's not rocket science.) Consult the scale! Sometimes we need to be more simple-minded. Isn't it much easier to weigh yourself to see if you're going in the right direction? Too often we would rather count calories than get on the scale—because the number on the scale is personal and can depress us or define us, if we let it. I don't recommend weighing after every meal, which is what I did at one time in my life, but I recommend checking in every now and then. Weighing yourself a couple of times weekly when you are trying to lose and once weekly when you are trying to maintain gives you a little reality.

And one more thing about the scale. Trusting without seeing will sometimes be required. I have had clients who did not see results for a week or two or who even went a little backward on the scale, but they finally experienced the fruits of change. I like what this passage says:

> Trust God from the bottom of your heart; don't try to figure out everything on your own. Listen for God's voice in everything you do, everywhere you go; he's the one who will keep you on track.[9]

I have a client right now who has lost some weight every week for six months. I'm pretty sure, based on experience, we will have a plateau at some point and will have to push through it. I'm expecting hardship, and yet I'm looking forward to ultimate victory as well.

KEEPING IT UP AND GETTING IT OFF

One of my challenges was pregnancy. The experts said a healthy weight gain was 25 to 35 pounds. The books said there was no need to gain in the last month. But I exceeded both of these and gained over 40 pounds by the time it was all said and done. It was painful to keep up healthy eating habits and consistent exercise only to be unpleasantly surprised by the number on the scale every time I stepped on. I was faithful to what I knew was the right approach, but it did not seem to be working for me at the time, which was frustrating.

My first baby weighed in at eight-and-a-half pounds, which explained some of the weight gain—and in the long run, persistence paid off. Not only did I have a beautiful and *healthy* baby, but the weight literally fell off afterward, revealing that there was a lot of baby and a whole lot of water. Working out and eating right throughout pregnancy actually did benefit my baby and my body, and sooner than expected I was wearing my pre-pregnancy clothes. So I encourage you also to do what is healthy and stick to it even if there are no immediate visible payoffs.

In the same way, it may take a while to reap the benefits of the new habits you have sown. We need a mentality overhaul, though, when it comes to food and weight loss. I purchased a cookbook last year entitled *Slow and Difficult Soups*. This provocative title resonated with me. (I suppose I could have titled this book *Slow and Difficult Weight Loss*, but I doubt the publishers would have gone for it.) But what I really want to drive home here is that the pounds you keep off are the ones you lose with hard work and patience. Long-term solutions can resolve long-term struggles. Expect to work—and expect to work at it for a long time. Some months the weight might melt off effortlessly, but other times it will feel like an uphill battle. However, you will get results and reach your goal if you persist. "Good things come to those who wait"—and in this case the wait is an active one!

Most of all, don't let yourself get discouraged along the way. Turn your eyes to God and receive the grace He offers, instead of looking at yourself and the failure and inadequacies you feel. When we pursue our goals, fixing our eyes on the Author and Perfecter of our faith, He comes through every time. Giving up dieting for the rest of our lives is so exciting! It makes me want to cheer for you, because I have been set free from the Diet Law, and I know the future joy, freedom, and leanness you will walk in!

MAKE IT
happen

Bury Idietry

1. Remember, change leads to freedom; rule-keeping leads to bondage.

2. Do not skip meals, cut out food groups, or count calories (oh yeah!).

3. Remember simplicity:
   Weight loss = energy burned > energy ingested

4. Weigh yourself in the morning, naked as a jaybird, and record your weight.

5. Weigh yourself one to three days a week as mentioned above.

6. Some weeks weight *maintenance* is a victory.

7. Persevere.

SALMON WITH SESAME SEEDS
Serves 4

4 small salmon fillets

¼ cup Bragg Liquid Aminos (a nutritious alternative to soy sauce)

3 tablespoons sesame seeds (I use dark ones)

2 teaspoons olive oil

1 teaspoon lemon juice

sea salt and freshly ground black pepper

In a large sealed plastic bag or shallow container, marinate the salmon fillets in the liquid aminos for 20 minutes. Preheat oven to 375°. Take salmon out of marinade and discard marinade. Spread sesame seeds onto a plate and roll the salmon in the seeds. Whisk olive oil and lemon juice together and drizzle on salmon pieces. Add a dash of sea salt and freshly ground pepper to each piece. Place salmon on a cookie sheet lined with foil for easy cleanup. Bake for about 15 minutes.

Salmon is a great source of omega-3 fatty acids and protein. It also boasts potassium, selenium, and vitamin B_{12}.

MIMI'S WHITE CHILI
Serves 8-10

1 pound dried large white beans, soaked overnight in water and drained

6-plus cups chicken broth

2-4 garlic cloves, minced

2 medium onions, chopped

1 tablespoon olive oil

2 4-ounce cans chopped green chilis

2 teaspoons ground cumin

1 ½ teaspoons dried oregano

¼ teaspoon cayenne pepper

4 cups cooked chicken breast (can boil 8 or so minutes to cook), diced

Combine beans, chicken broth, garlic, and half of the chopped onion in a large soup pot. Bring to a boil.

Reduce heat and simmer until beans are very soft (3 hours or more). Add more chicken broth if necessary. In a skillet, sauté remaining onion in oil until tender. Add chilis, cumin, oregano, and cayenne. Mix thoroughly.

Add to bean mixture. Add chicken and continue simmering 1 hour. Serve topped with grated cheese.

For a buffet, serve with some or all of the following toppings: chopped tomatoes, chopped parsley, chopped ripe olives, guacamole, chopped scallions, sour cream, crumbled blue-corn tortilla chips, shredded cheese, salsa. Cornbread makes a great addition to this meal.

Beans are one of the best weight-loss Super Foods (see chapter 9) because they are low in fat and a great source of complex carbohydrates and fiber. They are also loaded with antioxidants.

CHAPTER 4

KISS PERFECTION GOODBYE

Oh yes, you shaped me first inside, then out;
you formed me in my mother's womb.
I thank you, High God—you're breathtaking!
Body and soul, I am marvelously made!
I worship in adoration—what a creation!
You know me inside and out,
you know every bone in my body;
You know exactly how I was made, bit by bit,
how I was sculpted from nothing into something.

It seems like from the moment the doctor declares, "It's a girl!" we become contestants in a lifelong Barbie contest, whether we officially enter or not. Being born male still has its allowances for brawny, big, and tough, but being cut and ripped are increasingly more popular male ideals.

The pressure to conform to certain physical standards is felt by everyone here in the land of freedom, where life, liberty, and the pursuit of happiness are supposed to be our birthrights. We're not terribly free, though, and the pursuit of happiness is often eclipsed by or associated with the pursuit of thinness. We have all been impacted—some of us more than others—by those voices that whisper, "You're not thin enough," so pervasively that they can hound us to death.

So many of us want to buy the idea of quick weight loss no matter the cost. What compels us to go to extremes when it comes to weight loss? What drives us to try the absurd fads to the risky and dangerous weight-loss methods? What inspires us to put our faith in cellulite cream and even gastric (and drastic) bypass surgery and drugs? So many of us are willing to do whatever it takes to be more like Barbie or Ken.

Unreality Shows

Do we ever stop to think about the messages we are receiving, believing, and sometimes sending, or are we so brainwashed and blind-sighted that we no longer question reality? Speaking of which, do we really buy into the reality of so-called reality shows? I have four acquaintances who have been on what we could clearly call "unreality TV," two of whom are male models, and one of whom is a beauty queen, literally. The fourth one doesn't hold the titles, but she probably could have if she had pursued them. And these four have verified just how unreal most reality shows are.

Unreality is pitched to us in both subliminal and bold messages every single day. I was in the grocery store this morning to buy organic peanut butter and bread without high fructose corn syrup, and as the clerk was scanning my items I got bombarded with instant messages, not on my cell phone, but right in front of me on the shelves. Many of these magazine messages headlined were about outward appearance and the bod: "How to be Thin and Improve Your Skin"; "Bikini Body by June 1"; "Body Type Shopping Guide"; "Bye-Bye Flabby Thighs"; "Get Summer Sexy"; "Change Your Shape." One cover boasts a girl—all of 17 years old probably—showing off her hourglass figure. Another cover has a guy sporting his washboard abs. All are reminders that we either don't measure up…or that *we* measure *way up* on the scale. Their bodies are "perfect," making us green with envy, and there is a subconscious self-evaluation every time.

Torturously, the other magazine messages are all about food, glorious food, depicting scandalously cheesy casseroles, creamy pastas, and rich desserts. Some magazines go so far as to project a cover shot of a girl in an itsy-bitsy teeny-weeny yellow polka-dot bikini with an insert of a double-decker deliciously decadent devil's food cake, and the "recipe is quite simple really." What I want to know is, which recipe are they talking about—the one for the body or for the cake? Seriously, how can I have the cake (the body) and eat it (the cake) too? Both are gods of the day, and how cleverly pitted against each other. In reality, their incompatibility wreaks havoc. What an insidious tactic to hold us captive to self-indulgence, self-loathing, and self-sabotaging all at the same time!

Cultural emphasis on the body is relentless! We are blasted with images of the body via television, billboards, magazines, and movies, beginning at infancy. One message is inescapable: Your body should be beautiful and desirable, and here is the current standard. We don't stop to ponder why we should need a better body, because by the time we can reason, we have already been indoctrinated into the body philosophy of our culture: The body is a god—an object of worship. A perfect body equals a perfect life.

Never mind that each generation seems to laud a slightly different silhouette. Look at the contrast between the chubby arms, soft tummies, and modest breasts of the women portrayed in Renaissance paintings, versus the sculpted biceps, taut tummies, and buxom breasts of Hollywood's leading ladies today.

Unrealistic Bodies

The problem is, we don't stop to evaluate and distinguish truth from lies. Research confirms what we already know: "Ongoing exposure to certain ideas can shape and distort our perceptions of reality."[1] The sides of reality that we see have been airbrushed, plastified, and at the least worked on for hours by the hair and makeup crew. Whatever "reality" is left is completely unreal. Think about it: When do we most see unclothed or bathing-suited women? In the media, almost exclusively. The only time I see women unrobed in *real life* is in the Loehmann's public dressing area, and I admit, it's a dose of reality that is both shocking and relieving.

In 2002 Jamie Lee Curtis posed for *More* magazine just as she really is, sans touch-ups and refreshingly flawed. In the article called "True Thighs," she came out with this statement about the images of her body presented to the masses: "It's such a fraud. And I'm the one perpetuating it." One of her reasons for this bold display was to empathize with women who feel they don't measure up. The article goes on to say that the actress has struggled with feelings of inadequacy all her life and admits to trying it all, including plastic surgery. Thank you, Jamie Lee, for some reality from Hollywood.

We are constantly being beckoned to body worship, and, inevitably, we are getting unsolicited input about our own bodies and how they compare to the gold standard. From early childhood, we experience favor or disapproval based solely on appearance in some cases. Research affirms that criminals often get lighter sentences if they are "good-looking," and elementary school teachers often give special treatment to the pupils they think are "cute."[2] If we were to be honest, we have made some of these same biased judgments. And we seem to judge ourselves the most harshly.

∽∽∽∽

For most of us, namely women, it's like we're either overweight or weight-phobic. Whether we're eating as though we are a garbage disposal or we're wasting away on the latest diet, it's body abuse, plain and simple. Both gluttony and serious deprivation are expressions of a distorted view of the body. We tend to be lured by one of two major body extremes, which, working in tandem, set us up perfectly for one of the three diet traps.

Trap #1: We Strive for That Perfect Body

As a late bloomer by most counts, my girlish body matched up well to the images indelibly etched in my microchip through the age of 15. When my body began to morph into something more womanly, I remember feeling insecure. It was the early '80s, and extremely thin was "in." Flat was all that, and anorexia was *en vogue*...literally. In retrospect, we can point to numerous female celebrities who were blatantly struggling with body image. One of the most famous was songbird Karen Carpenter, who died from complications related to an eating disorder. The models of the day portrayed a bone-protruding thinness that seemed unattainable without a drastic restriction of calories.

My motivation for dieting was propelled by these countless photographs that had been burned on the pages of my mind, which created a certain orientation and expectation. I found that any variance from the so-called "it" body was intolerable to me. This presented a huge problem because I no longer mirrored the girlish body that epitomized beauty in the fashion magazines littering our coffee table at that time. I had been feeding myself a steady diet of *Seventeen* and *Glamour,* which exalted the emaciated body, while I simultaneously fed on junk food! When puberty hit me like a ton of doughnuts, it dealt a catastrophic blow to my world. Instead of embracing change and doing what I could to adjust my eating habits to an altered metabolism, I panicked and took the impetuous approach.

This impetuous approach was dieting. As I mentioned earlier, my dieting methods led to a nine-year detour down the dark path of disordered eating. I became a statistic for dieting taken to extremes. In chapter one, we briefly discussed the idea that eating disorders are fostered by diets. If you're in doubt, take a look at the following facts: In any six-month period, girls who diet severely are 18 times more likely to develop an eating disorder than non-dieters. Even moderate dieters are five times more likely to develop an eating disorder.[3] Let's face it, dieting contributes to disease and can even lead to death in some cases.

We can parallel our pursuit of "thin at all costs" to a popular sports mentality: "Win at all costs." Win at all costs for the athlete can mean playing a sport in spite of injury, using illegal and unhealthy ergogenic aids, or taking other drastic measures to enhance performance or increase the chances of winning. This phenomenon is becoming more and more common.

Why are we driven to these extreme pursuits? There is a strong belief system behind it all, and we must uproot it before it uproots us. This underlying system has one main premise: *The body is everything.* In other words, our bodies are all we have and all we *are,* often to the neglect of what lies beneath—our souls.

So if "the body is all we have," then a *perfected* body, of course, is our ultimate goal. And this is where the system starts to really break down because no matter how much we starve ourselves through dieting or carve ourselves through plastic surgery, the perfect body will always elude us. Instinctively, we know this, but we're not ready to own up to it yet, are we?

Why are we so excited to talk about the latest diet we are on, but take the discussion a bit deeper, to philosophical and spiritual beliefs about the body or identity issues, and that's getting way too personal? We'd rather just attach our identity to a number either on a scale or in a pants size. A number is tangible and, therefore, controllable, we think. And we're always eager for control.

Who's at the Center?

Really, our issue is one of idolatry. Idolatry simply means putting something else at the center of our lives instead of God. Let's return for a moment to that first act of rebellion that I mentioned. Our struggle with putting something else at the center began in the Garden. We see evidence of this "when she [Eve] saw that the fruit of the tree was good for food." In taking the forbidden fruit, she put her body before her devotion to God. This is often referred to as the lust of the flesh. But there was another factor in Eve's temptation that was more about the lust of the eyes: She saw that it was "pleasing to the eye and also desirable."[4] So the fruit not only answered a physical desire or hunger ("good for food"), but it was also physically attractive ("pleasing to the eye").

At that moment in time, Eve found herself consumed and captivated by a perceived physical need as well as a physical attraction. We can relate to her, as we have taken the cultural cues to value the physical—especially when it comes to our appearance—over everything else. It's scary the way Eve, after she had eaten something she knew she shouldn't have, suddenly felt the need to cover her naked body with fig leaves. Her immediate guilt manifested itself as shame of her body. Remember that they were first naked, and they felt *no* shame. Fig leaves, in this true story, are like the diets of today. We feel shame over the way our bodies look. After all, the body is everything, isn't it? So we panic and try to fix it quickly by grasping at something that might make us look better and feel more secure.

The story continues with Adam and Eve hearing God in the Garden and hiding. The answer to the problem of shame was, and still is for many of us, covering and hiding through dieting, makeup, the right clothes, the right look, breast implants, liposuction, lip collagen…. Like Adam and Eve, our self-consciousness and shame compel us to cover and hide. But what God desires most, and what we need most, is to come to Him. He is our hiding place and our covering. The most wonderful part of this story is when God provides garments of animal skin for them. This was the first of many sacrifices made on our behalf, up until that final sacrifice of His Son. This last act was more than enough to cover us, and yet all too often we still feel it's our job to cover ourselves.

In essence, the idolizing of beauty and the lie that the body is everything only leave us feeling unattractive, unloved, and unacceptable. Many of us are bound by another lie, which says that the body is nothing. And that leads us to trap number 2.

Trap #2: We Let Our Bodies Go

In *The Screwtape Letters,* C.S. Lewis uses dialogue between devilish beings to convey how dangerous it is when people view the body as inconsequential when compared with the spirit: "They constantly forget that whatever their bodies do affects their souls."[5]

A good number of those who don't subscribe to "the body is all" seem to just throw the body out with the bathwater instead. The idea that the body is nothing is all too common in some religious circles. Why? Because we know that the spirit matters so much! We're aware that God does not look at the same things as man does; for man looks at outward appearances but God looks at the heart.[6] God can actually *see* our hearts, which is sometimes a comforting thought and sometimes a scary one. So because of this, we often draw the extreme conclusion that our body is of no importance, and we pay no mind to what we look like. And in doing so, we disregard the outer expression of inner beauty that we were created to exude.

We begin to separate our bodies from our spirits in our philosophizing, and we buy wholeheartedly into the idea that "matter doesn't matter." This is a form of Gnosticism, a heretical movement of the latter part of the first century. Gnostic theology was dualistic, meaning that there is a supernatural realm and a natural realm, and the two should have nothing to do with one another. Some sects of Gnosticism actually taught that the material world was evil. If carried to an extreme, Gnosticism often leads to licentiousness. After all, if the body doesn't matter, then we can do whatever we want with it.

Separating the spiritual from the physical can lead us astray in a host of ways. One huge way would be how we care for the body—our eating and exercising habits. This idea that the body is nothing could manifest itself in overweight or obese tendencies. And ironically, as I will explain in more detail later, it could also be a forerunner to extreme dieting, nonnutritive eating, eating disorders, and sometimes it can even lead to death—the final blow to the body. Or it could rear its ugly head in other "body doesn't matter" habits, such as sexual promiscuity, smoking, alcoholism, drug abuse, inappropriate and revealing fashion choices, and, on the whole, a use of the body to manipulate any given situation or person.

The Extremes in Operation

When you are caught in the first trap—the body is everything—it often takes some bizarre twists and turns. What I have noticed is that sometimes an overemphasis on the *body* can eclipse attending to or caring about other external aspects. I have had the opportunity to consult with and, hopefully, help people on both sides of the weight coin (over and under weight), and I have often made this observation: Girls with eating disorders, such as anorexia and bulimia, are sometimes apathetic about makeup, hair, nails, what they wear, etc. If the body is what defines us, then we really need not concern ourselves with other outward details, right? Of course, another relevant reason for lack of self-care is a self-disdain, which is also prevalent in these cases. I think both are factors. I said this is an observation I've made, but it's also personal.

It hit me hard this past weekend. I was finishing a run at the local park, and I was about a mile from my car when I glanced at my watch. It was 11:30. I had that feeling sweep over me and that inner voice asking: *What am I forgetting?*... like in *Home Alone* when they are on the plane headed for Paris for the holidays, and the mom knows something's mysteriously off. She says: "I forgot something…did I turn off the coffee? Did you lock up? Did you close the garage? No that's not it…KEVIN!" Okay, so I'm thinking there's something I have to do…pick up the girls? Make a phone call? Turn in my latest writing installment…nope…WEDDING!

I realized that I was supposed to be at a wedding at 12:00 (in 30 minutes). I do the math: 8 minutes to my car, 10 minutes to my house, and 10 minutes to the wedding, assuming no roads are blocked off—an unsafe assumption in a city that has been under construction since the beginning of time, leaving me 2 minutes to get ready. I walked into the wedding at 11:58 (I'm not pretending I drove the speed limit) and, yes, I did have a cute dress and heels on, but you can imagine my hair!

The very next day, I'm getting ready for church and I forego the shower I didn't take the day before for the wedding. When I asked a good friend, "Does my hair look okay?" thinking it probably didn't look good but wanting reassurance that it did, I got an honest answer: "Not really." I wish I could say that I usually shower, fix my hair, shave my legs, paint my nails, and put on my makeup for church, special dates, speaking gigs and such, but it wouldn't be true. I am usually wearing jeans or workout clothes, a ponytail, and no makeup…all remnants of my old *body is everything* mentality. I usually leave little or no time for grooming, and I confess that I want to do better.

Now, I'm not implying that we should always look perfect. Perfectionism is a straitjacket. Besides, sometimes we really cannot spend time on our appearance because other things, like a sick spouse or a newborn or an 80-hour work week are all consuming, but, in general, we should do the best we can with what we've got and stop making excuses. And by the way, this includes every aspect of caring for our bodies, not just in terms of grooming.

Where's the Harmony?

All of us have pockets of incongruity in our lives. If you're married, your spouse has probably graciously (grin) brought them to your attention a time or two or ten, depending on how long you've been married. I'm talking about areas in which we don't live out what we know to be true—either subconsciously or consciously. This often happens when our spiritual and physical lives are not in harmony with one another.

For example, many of us have acquaintances who don't smoke or chew or go with guys or girls who do, nor do they drink to the point of drunkenness, and yet their eating habits are another story. The type and amount of "fuel" they ingest are completely out of balance with what their bodies require. These poor people are caught in the second trap, which says: "If the body is nothing, then it doesn't matter what or how much I put into it because *I* am not my body. In fact, I'm just going to ignore my body and my weight and eat whatever I want, whenever I want. I'm not going to concern myself with exercise or eating healthfully because those are bodily—insignificant—matters."

The reality is that the burden of being overweight affects much more than just our bodies. Here are some interesting findings which shed light on the ways in which the body and the psyche are related:

- "Overweight people are more likely to lose the weight and keep it off if they have a positive body image."[7]

- "Chronic dieters are much more likely than others to have a poor body image."[8]

- Women who received breast implants for cosmetic motivations, according to Finnish studies, were three times more likely to commit suicide than the general public.[9]

- "People who are satisfied with their bodies after a modest weight loss are more likely to keep the weight off."[10]

These are telling findings, friends.

Trap #3: We Waver Between Perfection and Permissiveness

Some of us live in trap one, where we are preoccupied with getting the perfect body, so we starve or we carve—if we have the cash. Others of us get ensnared by trap two, which says, "Oh, just forget the body. I'm much more than a biological being; I'm focusing on the development of the mind and soul." But I would venture to say that most of us live in trap three, which is somewhere in between. Sometimes we're striving for perfection, and sometimes we're just letting ourselves go. We live in the uncommitted middle, and dieting often seems to be the end result whichever way we lean.

Dieting is an obvious result of trap one because, in it, we're obsessed with our bodies. With its unpleasant and unhealthy rules and regulations, it can even be a way of punishing ourselves for not measuring up to the perfect image we have in our minds. And don't let trap two fool you. Its end result can often be dieting as well. Here is the progression: We keep telling ourselves that the body doesn't matter, then all of a sudden, after months or years of living this lie, we are overweight and exhausted, and it is negatively affecting everything we do. *Maybe the body does matter after all,* we realize. But by the time we wake up and smell the delusion, we are so enslaved by food, and exercise has become so foreign to our lethargic bodies, that losing weight the real (and slow) way seems impossible. Enter the latest "groundbreaking" diet, and we're hooked.

Trap three, a.k.a. the diet trap, is really all about weight cycling—we gain, we lose, we gain, we lose. We gain even more weight and then lose less. We read a book recommended by a friend because it "changed *her* life." We eat grapefruit for a month and lose some weight only to, as statistics confirm over and over, gain yet again.

In truth, the diet industry has had a field day with our wavering. And it has done its fair share of indoctrinating us with harmful ideas on the body and its purposes too. Our young people are being affected in more ways than we know. Here is a case in point: Researchers have dubbed the term "fat talk" to describe the way girls talk about their weight. Self-deprecating body talk is a form of bonding with their peers while avoiding deeper issues and feelings. They don't want to acknowledge or possibly don't know how to articulate their feelings of depression and dissatisfaction, so they resort to verbal body-bashing: "I'm so fat." This kind of talk can catalyze into full-blown eating disorders in particularly vulnerable girls. Really, it is a cry for reassurance, but body reassurance is not always the best answer because it emphasizes and directs even more focus to the body.[11]

Distorted body philosophies, like a tidal wave, can drown out self-value. And when that happens, our motives for losing those unwanted pounds are all wrong. We think once we reach our goal weight then our problems will be solved, but we couldn't be further from the truth. The right motivation must stem from the proper view of the body and its purposes. A healthy body image is a key component to our emotional and physical health, not to mention, our success in weight loss and maintenance. In other words, we must first get our heads on straight before we work on our bodies.

So how do we deal with these traps and all their pervasive lies? First, we need to admit our bondage. Next, we need to remember that the truth sets us free.[12] Clearly we must find out the truth about our bodies and how we should treat them, and in order to do this we need to understand God's take on our bodies. After all, He designed them.

Does God Like My Body?

Beauty comes in all different shapes and sizes and, therefore, we need to say adiós to Ken and Barbie. There is not one height, weight, and frame that comprise the most beautiful body type. We must stop believing the lies that we should or can have the perfect look. Actress Salma Hayek had something insightful to say about beauty: "People often say that beauty is in the eye of the beholder, and I say that the most liberating thing about beauty is realizing that you are the beholder. This empowers us to find beauty in places where others have not dared to look, including inside ourselves."

I'm not asserting that our physical appearance is equal to the inner person of the heart. If the outside matters, the inside matters more. The outward is a reflection of what we believe, value, and love.

That said, God created us with physical bodies. And the Bible says that they reflect His image in some way. "In His image" refers to mental, spiritual, and *bodily* reflection. The truth that we were made in the image of God gives sacredness, glory, and dignity to our bodies. In fact, the body has tremendous significance in Scripture, though we don't always ponder the depth of it.

First of all, look at the incarnation: God literally wrapped Himself in a human body: "And the Word became flesh and dwelt among us."[13] He lived on earth for 33 years in the tangible, even mortal, body of Jesus

Christ. Let that sink in a moment. The God of the universe chose to exist in a bodily form and die a physical death.

Secondly, Christ was resurrected in a bodily form as well. Remember that the disciples recognized Jesus, though for some, it took His showing them the scars in His hands and feet. When He rose from the dead, He had a new kind of body, a perfect body that was not subject to aging, weakness, or death. It was a body built for eternity. A perishable body was raised imperishable. A mortal body put on immortality. The apostle Paul points out that the resurrected body is a spiritual body, not meaning immaterial, but "suited to and responsive to the guidance of the Spirit."[14] We too will have a resurrected body, and many of us either forget or choose to forget this.

And thirdly, God chose to indwell our bodies when He sent His Spirit to live inside of us.[15] Did you catch that? Our bodies are miraculous containers of the Spirit of God. Our soul and spirit, along with God's Spirit will reside in our bodies until we graduate from this life. And then, as we just saw, we will have a new, resurrected, physical body that houses who and what we are for eternity. Whew! These are mysterious realities, but they should answer something we often wonder: Does God like my body? Clearly, He does.

Does God Want *Me* to Like My Body?

So what *does* God desire when it comes to how we see our bodies? I believe we can take a lesson from my youngest. My precious five-year-old was about to hop in the shower one day when she made this proclamation: "Mommy, I think my body is beautiful." It was not based on vanity or society's definition of a beautiful body, for she was still naive to cultural standards of beauty. Rather, it was based on her delight in the "wonder" of her body—a love and acceptance of how God made her. (In fact, she was so comfortable in her body that she saw no need for clothes for the first four years of her life.)

I may never hear such pure words regarding a naked body again. I wish I could shelter her from having to struggle with her body image as she gets older, but I'm afraid that's not realistic. I can, however, model and reflect back to her an honor toward my own body and hers. I am teaching her how to care for and nurture her body through nutrition, movement, and stewardship of her athleticism and one day…when she forgets…I will remind her that she is fearfully and wonderfully made.

It takes some heavy-duty armor to shield ourselves from the lies of culture, to be sure. I believe that acquiring a scriptural perspective is essential. We must constantly renew our minds and strive to apply a God-like grid. Will we, like David, look in the mirror and say, "I am fearfully and wonderfully made"?

Sometimes choosing to see beauty based on what we know rather than what we may actually *see* at first will be required. But if we choose God's view—that our bodies are good—consistently, we will begin to own it. Eventually, we will grow to have a heart of thankfulness, love, and gratitude for our bodies. God already thinks you are beautiful, and He wants you to agree with Him and praise Him for it.

Although we can look at our society and see contradictions to this, St. Paul said no one ever hated his own body, and I think I get the point. The implication is that we have every reason to nurture and care for our bodies. Seriously, how bizarre is it to hate our bodies anyway! We should be fueling them with nutrient-dense food so that they will thrive. Eating healthfully is responsible stewardship of this wonderfully intricate body we're given. And we must exercise our bodies so that they might not be a hindrance but a partner to the Spirit that lives inside us.

This is so that we can fulfill our purposes on this earth with energy and strength, training the body to be a strong and healthy for the work of the Lord. We are called to assist and serve those around us. Don't you think having a healthy body would be beneficial in this? Furthermore, everything we do is supposed to glorify God. Well, if everything we do is done in the body, that means all our resting, playing, walking, running, singing, laughing, making love in the context of marriage…everything we do can be a part of fulfilling our highest calling—to reflect God's glory.

Do you see it? The way we treat our bodies is another way we fulfill our ultimate purpose. *So where do we start?* you may be wondering. We start by kissing perfection goodbye. Let's look at two ways we can do this.

1. Get a New Bodytude

No doubt, putting the body in proper perspective in a world where it is worshipped is a daunting and ongoing task. In fact, it's impossible without divine intervention. God in His mercy revealed to me that I was allowing the culture to define not only the silhouette of the ideal body but the purpose of the body as primarily an object of beauty. It took time and prayer to change my bodytude. Prior to this change, I had never understood that eating healthy was spiritually relevant.

Getting a spiritual grip on the purpose and design of my own body changed and continues to impact my life! Once I made a commitment to treat my body like God's house, there was no place for dieting. Dieting had revealed the incongruity between how I fed my body and how I fed my spirit. I was uncomfortable in my own skin, and it distracted me from loving and serving God with my whole being.

On the other hand, when we are self-controlled, respectful, and honoring of the body, we worry less about what others think about our appearance and focus on just loving them.

2. Meditate on the Truth That Sets You Free

The spiritual discipline of meditation has fallen on hard times through the years. Some picture sitting in a room with their legs crossed, chanting for thirty minutes while others imagine catching some zzz's. Actually, meditation is a good thing, and not only is it recommended by renowned psychologists, but it is also encouraged in the Bible. To meditate means "to chew the cud," like a cow ruminates its food in order to reap more benefits from it.

We need to steep ourselves in the truth. Take a look at some Bible verses that speak directly about the body and its purposes.* There are so many. Read them. Meditate on them. Pray them into your very being...own them.

Personally, my favorite body verse is Romans 12:1, which I recite every time I speak on the body. It says: "I urge you, brethren, by the mercies of God, to present your bodies a living and holy sacrifice, acceptable to God, which is your spiritual service of worship."[16] *The Message* translates it this way: "So here's what I want you to do, God helping you: Take

---

* For example, Genesis 1:27,31; Psalm 139:13-16; Romans 6:19-20; 2 Corinthians 4:7; 7:1).

your everyday, ordinary life—your sleeping, eating, going-to-work, and walking-around life—and place it before God as an offering."

Our everyday, bodily life matters to God, as it is an opportunity for worship. Take a look at this passage: "We have this treasure in earthen vessels."[17] It points to the significance of our bodies—we are both containers of immense spiritual treasure, yet we are also imperfect, or *earthenly,* if you will. The verse prior to this says that God gave us the light of the knowledge of the glory of God in the face of Christ. Though this is a somewhat lofty verse to understand, we can establish that God's glory was manifested in the physical body of Jesus Christ. By the same token, our physical bodies also reflect God's glory, as we touched on earlier.

<center>~~~~~</center>

We can exalt the body and give it power, mystique, and priority that it doesn't deserve, and we can also diminish the importance of the body, saying that it has no relevance for us as spiritual beings. In other words, we can overemphasize the body or trivialize it.

Or we can try to find balance in the pursuit of spiritual and physical harmony. Our goal in desiring to lose weight and live lean should stem from an integration of the two. In other words, we must bridge the disconnect between body and spirit and examine our motives and our approach to weight loss. Here are some helpful questions to ask ourselves during the process: Is the emphasis on beauty or on being good stewards with what we've been given? Is our weight loss motivated by perfecting the outer shell or by gaining freedom from enslavement to it? The latter in both instances goes deeper and will keep us tracking long after the beauty has faded. Now, is our weight loss driven by a desire to look good or to be healthy, or both? I think these two go hand in hand, and that's okay. Remember my little girl who took delight in her beautiful body?

If you chose the latter every time, then you are ready to embrace change, quit the dieting game, and accept a new bodytude. Okay, let's get on with some highly practical applications leading to weight loss. Let's get losing!

MAKE IT
happen

Let's Get Physical and *Spiritual!*

1. Pay attention and analyze the cultural messages you are receiving about the body.

2. Pray that God would help you see yourself as He does.

3. Get in front of a mirror and recite this motto—"I am fearfully and wonderfully made"—daily, until you accept it.

4. Meditate on Scripture that puts the body into a biblically correct paradigm.

5. Be a role model to friends, children, and others. Our body acceptance can have a positive impact on those around us.

6. Analyze your motivations for weight loss, viewing weight loss as an act of stewardship rather than a requirement for acceptance.

7. Focus on health and a healthy weight, which expresses care for the body, rather than focusing on imperfections of self.

8. Work on the things that are in your control. For example, your height is out of your control. You can establish a normal, healthy, desirable weight for your frame and body type by implementing the strategies in the next chapters.

9. A practical piece of advice that I try to abide by is to keep from purchasing and displaying pictures of scantily clad models selling the perfect body. Protect yourself, your spouse, and your children from this form of instant messaging.

CANDY BAR ALTERNATIVE
Serves 7

1 cup almonds

½ cup pecans or pecan pieces

¼ cup dark chocolate chips

Mix ingredients together. Scoop out in ¼-cup servings (there should be about 7) and put into small containers or baggies for occasional "on the go" snacks or for when you crave chocolate. Sometimes I put these in lunch boxes for a treat. You can store these snacks in the freezer for several weeks.

Almonds are calorie and nutrient-dense, which is why these servings are small. They are an excellent source of monounsaturated and polyunsaturated (both good) fats. They are also a good source of protein, potassium, calcium, and iron.

Dark chocolate, though high in fat, is a good source of antioxidants and flavonoids, which are plant pigments that have a host of health benefits. Think moderation.

CHAPTER 5

KISS THE COUCH GOODBYE

> **Lack of activity destroys the good condition of every human being, while movement and methodical physical exercise save it and preserve it.**
>
> *—Plato*

Recently I had the privilege of going to Israel with a group of over 200 people of all different ages. The trip was an absolute delight. The sightseeing and biblical history were both breathtaking and fascinating.

Each day we took a tour bus to a historical site. We did our fair share of walking to and from the bus, and one would assume that we were getting plenty of exercise, but in reality, much of the day was spent standing and listening to explanations about the archaeological site and then meandering over to the next ruin. Couple this with the fact that there was amazing food everywhere we turned, and you can guess what happened: caloric input was outweighing energy expenditure

The traditional Middle-Eastern offerings—including hummus, falafel (which consist mainly of fried fava beans or chickpeas), baba ghanoush (an eggplant and sesame seed mixture similar to hummus), feta cheese, and olives—were in abundance, not to mention the fact that they're also highly abundant in fat. Toward the end of the ten days, I heard quite a few commenting that clothes were fitting *snuggish* and that they were feeling a bit *sluggish*—telltale signs of weight gain.

Though the lean choices were limited, I enjoyed the food immensely, especially the fresh yogurt, fish, and hummus. Daily I compromised my good food habits with whole-fat dairy products and buffet-style eating. Yet when I returned home, one of my girlfriends made the comment that I looked like I had lost some weight. In fact, I discovered that I had lost two pounds when I got on the scale to see. And I didn't even avoid sauces, ban chocolate, or skip meals. (It's against my modus operandi!)

You see, every time I have a break in my normal routine, such as vacations or trips, birthday parties, holidays, special occasions, I have the intention of staying close to my ideal weight. Because in the real world—as opposed to the diet world, where you are expected to special order or carry your frozen Jenny Craig food with you everywhere you go—the food choices set before us are often out of our control. So it's up to us to exercise what *is* in our control. Truthfully, I do splurge during these special times, and yet I still fit into *most* of my jeans—we all have a pair of "skinny" jeans that fit about 10 out of 365 days, right? Want to know my secret? It's what's helped me to lose those extra pounds and never find them again. But before I tell you, you'll have to stop flirting with some faulty concepts.

Kiss the French Lady Goodbye

Perhaps you have read the clever and refreshing book *French Women Don't Get Fat,* by Mireille Guiliano. In it, she reveals *her* secret to success when it comes to staying slender and svelte. Her main focus is on lifestyle activity, a concept that has been touted frequently in health magazines and online articles. It's the idea that we can get all the exercise we need by simply incorporating more physical activity into our daily lives, via walking places, taking the stairs when we have the option, parking further away when we drive somewhere, and so on.

I agree that lifestyle activity qualifies as part of the fit equation, and I will devote a chapter to this; however, relying on it as our sole means of exercise is a flawed concept. We just won't get enough of it. Unless you live in a city like New York or Paris, walking to the market, shops, and restaurants is not an option. Walking is trés chic as well as trés practical in a few select cities around the world. However, those of us who reside outside these cities need not let our naïveté get the best of us. Let's face it, walking to the market means one or more of the following: walking much of the way over and under dangerous freeways, getting attacked by ferocious dogs, getting accosted by street dwellers, and quite possibly having a heat stroke before arriving at our intended destination.

And furthermore, we live in a convenience-driven, fast-paced society that makes it nearly impossible for us not to fall in line and rely on those conveniences daily. As much as I will urge you to rethink these patterns, chances are the car, elevator, escalator, and moving sidewalk will often win out over walking.

It's true it wasn't always this way. Think about the amount of exercise necessary for living and spreading the gospel during the time of Christ and His disciples. They walked hundreds of miles some weeks in order to carry out their mission and full-time occupation. Christ was never portrayed to be in a hurry, but He certainly had places to go, people to heal, miracles to perform, and the very words of God to deliver. In one compelling article, the author concluded that Jesus would have walked a grand total of 21,525 miles on trips taken during his 33 years on this earth. By the way, the distance around the world at the equator is 24,901.55 miles (40,074 km). Mary, His mother, walked about half the distance around the world on trips by the time she was 50 years old![1]

The great treks people in past cultures purposefully took qualified as aerobic activity. *Aerobic* simply means "with oxygen," and aerobic exercise involves some form of continuous, rhythmic activity using the large muscle groups.

In fact, aerobic, or cardiovascular, exercise—terms I will use interchangeably—could mostly be achieved through walking in American cities up until the early 1900s, when Henry Ford's new and improved conveyor belt–based assembly line came on the scene. By 1927, 15 million Model Ts had been manufactured. Shortly thereafter, people started building cities for cars, not for walking. There are occasional exceptions, but nowadays we rarely *need* to walk anywhere.

Here is an example of one of those exceptions: In the aftermath of Hurricane Katrina, our church was in charge of coordinating the interfaith relief efforts of feeding, serving, and helping the thousands of New Orleans evacuees at the George R. Brown Convention Center in Houston. During the week I volunteered, I walked across a 1.2-million-square-foot building numerous times, carrying strollers, babies, and children. This wasn't your moderate-paced kind of walking; it was some serious and purposeful walking. Rare days like these are some of the very few in my life that I get sufficient exercise without setting apart a specific time for it.

Unfortunately, general lifestyle movement usually won't cut the Dijon when it comes to burning calories. We need to raise our heart rate for a continuous 20 minutes in order to burn fat, and most lifestyle activity barely makes us break a sweat. The idea that a leisurely stroll will help us lose weight is really an insult to our common sense, because instinctively we know that intensity matters.

Burn More Calories Than You Eat

After examining the failure rate and the distorted views of the body implicit in dieting, my hope was to convince you that the only way to lose weight *permanently* is to change our minds and our habits. Changing our minds and habits, in this case, involves swimming upstream a little bit. When it comes to Weight Loss 101, the goal is to expend more than you take in. In other words, you have to burn more calories than you eat. Some people would say it is eating less calories than you burn. Do you see the difference? It may be subtle, but the implications are huge.

The fact is, our society is more sedentary and bigger than ever, and yet diet plans bombard us every which way. Studies are showing that we are actually consuming less fat and less overall calories than 20 years ago, and yet we are still gaining girth. Maybe we should address the other half of the glass…perhaps the answer isn't in being empty, so to speak.

Truth is, the glass is half full—of exercise. We need a program that puts *at least* half of the emphasis on consistent cardiovascular exercise and less emphasis on restricting our caloric intake. Losing weight—or burning fat—requires what you may have suspected: regular rigorous exercise.

Researchers at Duke University Medical Center separated 175 over-weight middle-aged men and women into three groups: One group was assigned the task of walking or jogging 11 miles weekly; another group was assigned the task of jogging 17 miles weekly; and the third group continued their usual lifestyle. At around the six-month mark, the 17-mile joggers lost almost 11 pounds of fat. The walk/jog 11 miles group lost about 4.5 pounds of fat (walkers) or 6 pounds of fat (joggers). Guess what? The non-exercisers gained about 2.5 pounds of fat. Notice, this study mentions nothing regarding their diets but deals solely with exercise.

"In most people who are overweight, it's a slow but steady gain of one to five pounds over the course of the year," says Duke's Cris Slentz, an exercise physiologist who coauthored the study.[2] This slow-gaining phenomenon is not because we start eating more and more annually but because with each year our metabolism slows down and we lose muscle mass if we do not exercise. By the same token, regular exercise gets our metabolisms stoked for fat burning both now and later. And, as an added benefit, the more intense we make our workouts, the more fired up our metabolisms get. Remember, intensity matters, and the Duke study affirms this. Why does intensity matter? Here are the two main reasons: 1) Our time is limited, and, therefore, burning more calories in a shorter amount of time is advantageous. And 2) intensity has long-term benefits for our metabolism.

In summary, consistent cardiovascular exercise is crucial to perma-nent fat loss. Here's how it works: Take an average guy during inactivity. He may burn 60 to 70 calories per hour. Now, take that same person and measure caloric expenditure during a *sustained, high-level* activity (rapid walking, running, swimming, or bicycling would qualify), and it could reach 1000 calories per hour. Impressive math, even for someone who is already convinced that continuous, sustained, aerobic exercise pays big calorie-burning dividends.

Now, let's put our guy on a two-miles-a-day jogging program, and he will use up about 6000 calories in a month, accounting for about 2 pounds of fat. It doesn't take an astrophysicist to calculate the number for six months and come up with 12 pounds of fat, gone!

Here is another fact you might find interesting: If you have pounds to lose, the excess weight you carry will cause you to burn *more* calories for the same amount of exercise than the skinny guy on the EFX next to you. How is this possible? You expend more energy by moving more weight, and you end up losing more fat in the long haul. This is not an excuse to stay overweight but a motivation to get going.

Before we move on, chew on this for a moment: Endurance athletes, such as Lance Armstrong (and any other "Tour de Francer") or ultra-distance runners, sometimes consume between 6000 and 13,000 calories per day.[3] Are you starting to see that being "full" isn't our biggest foe?

The Most Significant Factor in Weight Loss

Well, now that we've exposed some faulty concepts when it comes to consuming and burning calories, you can probably guess what keeps me from experiencing the typical post-trip scale shock. It's regular exercise…yes, even in Israel.

When I arrived at the hotels in Jerusalem and Tiberius, I inquired about safe jogging routes, fitness equipment, and exercise classes. I covered my blonde hair with a cap and jogged a three-mile-out-and-back route from our hotel when I could get myself out of bed. Instead of taking the elevator, I power-walked the snake path up to the great Herodian fortress of Masada. And I was noticeably the only Gentile in a highly choreographed aerobics class cued in Hebrew.

You get the picture. People who want to become leaner have to get up and move. There are lots of negotiables in my weight-loss methodology, but consistent cardiovascular exercise is not one of them! In fact, consistency in exercise paves the way for negotiation in other areas of lean living—great news for chocoholics!

There have been studies citing that restricting calories does lead to weight loss. In the follow-up studies, however, research confirms that calorie restriction alone does not, I repeat, *does not* lead to *permanent* weight loss. Up to 95 percent of dieters return to their original weight or even add pounds.

Unlike the conflicting nature of diets—protein versus carbs, fat versus sugar—there is really no debate about exercise. Everyone is confirming that exercise is the most significant factor in lasting weight loss. In a recent *Consumer Reports* research study, regular exercise was the number one successful weight-loss maintenance strategy. Eighty-one percent of the successful participants in the study cited exercise as their primary tactic.

As I look around, the people I know who are always trying the latest diet are not the ones who exercise regularly, so it should come as no surprise that they're losing in the long-term fight against fat. They are the ones taking one step forward and two steps backward. Truth be told, when someone loses weight through a diet without exercise, I hold the applause. Though I'd never want to see anyone fail, I can't help but count the days until the pounds start creeping up on them. I know it sounds skeptical, but I have simply observed the reality of the failure rate.

On the other hand, when people lose weight through consistent exercise and changing their nutrition habits, I can rejoice with them in good faith. A lady on our church staff lost over 80 pounds ten years ago, and she has kept it all off. Her secret? She will tell you that exercise changed her life. Successful "losers" have discovered exercise, and they won't stop till they drop.

A few years ago, Janice, a stay-at-home mom whose boys were in high school at the time, came to me with a desire to lose about ten pounds and to increase her lean muscle mass. She claimed to have never been very athletic, which was about to change. Over the course of about ten weeks of training she took off most of the weight, and as a bonus she took years off of her appearance, which is often an added benefit of losing weight through exercising. Something else happened to Janice. She got pumped about working out, and in her mid-40s, she became a certified group-exercise instructor. She has kept the weight off, and she now teaches a mean spinning class weekly.

The people I have trained, the regulars in my various exercise classes over the years, the friends I run with, those I see frequently at Memorial Park (my third home and a three-mile wooded loop in Houston), all have one thing in common: They are all cardio crazed because they know that cardiovascular exercise is the most efficient, rational, inexpensive, and often downright enjoyable weapon in the battle of the bulge.

Just as daily prayer and the reading of God's Word are foundational to spiritual health, so is consistent cardio to permanent weight loss. For those of us who have desired a thriving relationship with God while neglecting the basics, we understand that it sometimes takes spiritual frustration to get us to do the obvious. Many of you reading this are thinking that exercise sounds so simple and obvious, but have you gotten frustrated enough to finally buckle down and do it?

The truth is that most people aren't doing it, and the rest aren't doing enough of it. Only 15 percent of Americans work out vigorously at least three times a week.[4] We are a couch-potato nation that is focused on cutting out the potato when, in actuality, what we need most is to get up off the couch.

Are You Floating in Denial?

One of the questions I ask my husband monthly is, "Sweetheart," (because he is most of the time) "what am I in denial about?" I have lived long enough to realize that everyone is in denial about something. I have met melancholy people who actually think they are sanguine and vice versa. Some of us live in absolute denial, and others of us just need a good reality check every now and then.

One thing I have noticed as a weight-loss advisor and personal trainer over the past decade is that the majority of people are in severe denial about the number of sedentary hours in their days. We like to think we are fairly active people. We think that we are active enough because we A) live on the second floor of an apartment complex and take the stairs daily B) walk Fido around the block in the AM and PM C) walk to the break room, water cooler and, therefore, the loo frequently. In our minds we are burning some serious calories. The fact is we are doing very little.

Our caloric intake well outweighs the caloric expenditure of everyday activity because we're competing with so much everyday *in*activity, including the TV (and accompanying remote) and the computer. Unless you are one of the elite professional athletes in this country or a mom with several children under the age of six who doesn't "do" fast food, which is becoming an oxymoron, your desk job plus your gum chewing aren't cutting it in the calorie-burning department.

The Amazing Benefits of Exercise

Perhaps you aren't living in denial and you are convinced that exercise is the best way to lose weight, but you need just a little more prodding to get started. Let's look at some of the positives of exercise. Here are just a few of its amazing benefits:

1. improving the metabolism
2. protecting the heart
3. improving digestion
4. prolonging life
5. protecting against some forms of cancer
6. reducing the risk of dementia
7. combating depression
8. improving sleep
9. minimizing menopausal symptoms
10. protecting men's sexual and urinary health

Exercise is also something you do as opposed to do without, which has many positive ramifications. And another great thing about it is that exercise can be addressed in a short time slot in our day. Dieting, on the other hand, must be revisited every time we think about putting something in our mouths. Exercise is freeing. Dieting is limiting. Exercise is something we can incorporate indefinitely. Dieting, because of its super-strict nature, is temporary. Exercise is your friend—dieting, your foe!

We've touched on the health and weight-loss benefits of exercise, but there's more! Exercise is a great way to reduce stress and clear your head. Many people feel relaxed and relieved after an exercise session.[5] It's a time to leave corporate pressures behind and break from the demands to serve, produce, and earn our keep. When I had a newborn baby (both times), exercise was about mental survival. It also has been shown to boost social confidence, as well as naturally enhance mood through the release of endorphins.

Probably one of the biggest benefits of exercise, however, is one of the main mottos of this book: Exercise covers a multitude of sins. (Hey, that would be a good book title.) I repeat this phrase to clients often so that it will be indelibly etched in their brains. Now, I don't mean to imply that exercise can atone for kicking the neighbor's dog, but rather, in the area of weight loss, exercise covers a multitude of high calorie indulgences, faux pas, and compromises. The temptation to overeat is consistently before us, and, simply put, exercise should be just as consistent.

Getting Started

When someone asks me, "What is the best cardiovascular exercise for weight loss?" as partial as I am to running, my response is, "The one you will do!" For some ideas, see the chart below (developed by the American College of Sports Medicine) for calories burned per hour of various exercise modes:

Activity (1 hour)	Calories burned based on your body weight		
	130 lbs	155 lbs	190 lbs
Aerobics, general	354	422	518
Bicycling, 12-14 mph, moderate	472	563	690
Dancing, aerobic, ballet, modern	354	422	518
Judo, karate, kick boxing, tae kwan do	590	704	863
Race walking	384	457	561
Rollerblading	413	493	604
Rope jumping	590	704	863
Running, 6 mph (10 min mile)	590	704	863
Running, 6.7 mph (9 min mile)	649	774	949
Running, 7 mph (8.5 min mile)	679	809	992
Running, treadmill	472	563	690
Running, upstairs	885	1056	1294

Skiing, cross-country, moderate effort	472	563	690
Skiing, downhill, moderate effort	354	422	518
Stairmaster	354	422	518
Swimming laps, fast	590	704	863
Swimming laps, moderate effort	472	563	690
Walking, 3.0 mph, moderate pace	207	246	302
Walking, 4.0 mph, very brisk pace	236	281	345
Water aerobics, water calisthenics	236	281	345

Some studies show that people tend to exercise longer and feel more satisfied when an activity goes with their personality.[6] How much, how hard, and how often? I'm so glad you asked. I have mapped out for you some detailed exercise guidelines for optimal weight loss in chapter 12.

Instead of overwhelming you with an impressively complicated prescription, I have a *Keep It Simple, Sweetie* plan. Simplicity is a huge part of my exercise and eating well philosophy. The main components of this weight-loss program include cardiovascular exercise + quality control and portion control in relation to food + strength training + prayer, which can be remembered by my acrostic KISS. KISS, in this plan, stands for Kardio, Intake, Strength, and Spirit. If you are eager to make it happen, skip ahead in chapter 12 and come back to chapter 6 for the rest of the story. In the meantime, see the following pointers on how to make consistent exercise a reality in your life.

MAKE IT
happen

Ten Ways to Get Gritty About Exercise

1. Pray for God's help as you commit to exercising for life.

2. Find an exercise friend or a group to exercise with.

3. Set realistic goals, write them down, and share them with someone else.

4. Experiment with different activities and find what fits your personality and preferences.

5. Reward yourself with non-food pleasures for keeping your exercise goals: Schedule a massage or a pedicure, sleep in one day, allow yourself an hour of reading time in front of the fireplace with herbal tea, take a bubble bath, subscribe to a healthy-cooking magazine, get a new multitasking workout outfit.

6. Find a walk/run trail, join a nearby gym, buy a piece of cardio equipment or a bike.

7. Combine exercise with something you love. For me, it's being outdoors. For you, it could be doing the treadmill while watching your favorite show, or listening to your tunes or a book on CD, or power-walking while you memorize Scripture or pray, or bringing your baby in the jogger—both of my girls thought this was a delight until they started walking, or bringing your beloved dog. This way, it's so enjoyable that you miss it if you don't do it.

8. If you are on a tight, inflexible schedule, plan the time of day you will exercise and put it in your PDA.

9. Keep an exercise journal for one month so that you can observe your faithfulness.

10. Hire a certified personal trainer for a few sessions or until you reach your goal weight.

QUINOA AND OATS BREAKFAST PORRIDGE
Serves 4

3 cups water

¼ teaspoon salt

¼ cup quinoa (pronounced keen-wah)

1 cup oats

½ teaspoon cinnamon

2 teaspoons vanilla

2 tablespoons maple syrup or honey

¼ heaping cup of walnut pieces or pecan pieces (I often mix them)

¼ cup of dried cranberries or chopped dates

In a medium pot bring water and salt to a boil. Add quinoa, reduce heat, and simmer for about 7 minutes. Add oats and simmer another 7 minutes until liquid is absorbed and porridge thickens (stirring as it thickens). Add the rest of the ingredients and stir for 1 minute. Serve with a little milk or a tablespoon of cream per bowl.

This is a hearty, feed-your-body-well kind of breakfast. It is a good pre-workout meal because it has a nice balance of the macronutrients. If you are making it for one, it keeps well for 4-5 days in the fridge (I mix the nuts in just before eating this if I am saving some). Just reheat and you have several days of a home-cooked breakfast.

I eat this most winter mornings.

Key nutrients:

Oats have been getting great press. They are cholesterol lowering and they contain the (good for you) polyunsaturated fatty acids. Oats are a good source of soluble fiber, magnesium, and iron.

Quinoa is a fantastic source of protein because it contains all of the essential amino acids and is one of the least allergenic grains. Not only is it a fine protein source, it boasts a good amount of magnesium and manganese and healthy levels of B_2, E, and fiber. It contains iron, copper, phosphorus, and zinc.

CHAPTER SIX

KISS FLAB GOODBYE

**She sets about her work vigorously;
her arms are strong for her tasks...
She is clothed with strength and dignity;
she can laugh at the days to come.**

Like many old-fashioned women who perceive themselves to be modern, I was a bit skeptical about women benefiting from strength training or working the muscles against some kind of resistance, such as weights. I didn't want to "bulk up" and look like a WWF wrestler. I wanted to lean down. My husband, Ben, tried to convince me that I wouldn't necessarily get bigger, but I couldn't be persuaded by an ectomorph (naturally svelte body type) to weight-train. I had visions of my mesomorphic body (naturally muscular body type) becoming hulkomorphic (imaginary body type) if I worked out with weights.

There are actually three general body types: *ectomorph, mesomorph,* and *endomorph.* (Endomorphs tend to be the round and soft types.) Ben credited weight training for the physical transformation he underwent his freshman year in college, going from a self-proclaimed awkward, skinny guy to the strong, lean, and muscular guy I fell head over heels in love with. Finally, I took my husband's advice and consented to trying it. (In actuality, I came across some convincing research in a reputable exercise journal, but he doesn't have to know that.)

BODY TYPE CATEGORIES

Ectomorph—generally lean and lightly muscled, think an NBA player.

Endomorph—usually short but thick limbs and heavy bones, think NFL defensive lineman.

Mesomorph—tends to be muscular, athletic, and lean.

Though some people are purely *ecto, endo,* or *meso,* frequently people will fall into mixed categories, such as ecto-mesomorphs.

Much to my surprise, without even trying to lose fat by adding more Kardio (cardiovascular exercise) or cutting out calories, my body composition favorably changed. While we don't choose where we lose (spot reduction is as mythical as middle-age spread, which we will touch on in the following paragraphs), we *can* actually build up certain body parts. Weight training has the advantage of helping to reshape the body no matter what your body type. Our genetics cannot be changed, but we can work with what we have. Within reach of my weight-loss goal, I lost the last few pounds and dropped a pant size effortlessly after getting consistent with weight training.

After several months of lifting weights, I discovered an added benefit to my newfound routine—I was getting stronger. I went from thinking dips, an exercise in which the upper body has to support and lift the whole body over a short distance, were impossible for females, to completing eight repetitions one day. I was later humbled to discover that some girls can actually do chin-ups too, which requires even more upper body strength.

Stronger muscles also add to our everyday quality of life, especially if you have a lot of heavy lifting as part of your daily routine associated with the likes of young children, aging parents, frequent travel, or even a physically challenging job such as physical therapy. The biblical superwoman role model described in Proverbs 31 was strong: "She girds herself with strength [spiritual, mental, and physical fitness for her God-given task] and makes her arms strong and firm."[1] We can be inspired by her example of strength for her tasks. Why should we dread carrying luggage through an airport, hauling groceries upstairs, getting the 30-pound bag of dog food out of the car, or even hauling junior in his baby carrier to grandma's house? Common chores become less strenuous when we are strong, fit, and confident.

Weight Training Helps You Shed the Pounds

We've established that cardiovascular exercise is a critical key to long-term weight loss. Strength training is another important piece of the puzzle. Strength training builds muscle, which is going to help you lose weight and maintain your goal weight. More muscles actually utilize more calories even at rest. This means that a muscular person, even while sleeping, is burning more calories than their non-muscular counterpart because muscle is more metabolically active than fat. For every pound of muscle gained you will burn more calories per day. The bottom line is that you can gain strength and lose fat with weight training.

In a 12-week study involving a strength-training regimen, subjects increased their strength anywhere from 24 percent to 92 percent and their body fat decreased by 3 percent. Their muscles became more active metabolically and therefore increased resting metabolic rate (RMR) by an average of 8 percent RMR. RMR is the minimum number of calories your body needs to support its basic physiological functions such as breathing and circulating blood. This translated to the consuming of 300 extra calories a day, much more than the actual exercise itself burned, to maintain their weight (this was not a weight-loss study but the ramifications are hugely applicable). Had calories been reduced, obviously they would have lost weight.[2] By the way, your RMR is one of the primary contributors to energy expenditure (70 percent).

RATING YOUR METABOLISM

Your metabolic rate =
your resting metabolic rate + energy consumed by daily activities

Things that affect your metabolic rate:

1. *Muscle*—more muscle increases your RMR.
2. *Age*—your RMR tends to decrease with age.
3. *Weather*—living in a cold climate can increase RMR.
4. *Meals*—small regular meals will increase your RMR.
5. *Crash dieting*—it will *decrease* your RMR.

Before progress "blessed us" with so many modern conveniences, men and women got plenty of muscle-moving opportunities simply based on daily necessities. Food preparation was a constant and laborious effort which included grinding flour, planting and picking fruits and veggies off the vines, carrying them, and cooking over an open fire, and let's not forget cutting, gathering, and hauling the firewood. In some developing countries, where obesity and overweight populations are rare, manual labor is still a part of their culture even among the wealthy. I was able to experience this myself when I worked with an international organization called Youth With A Mission after I graduated from college. During a two-month outreach to Mexico, I quickly became accustomed to the manual labor required for daily functionality. After accomplishing labor-intensive chores such as washing clothes on a washboard, I gained a new appreciation for the technology and gadgetry that are standard household appliances and time-saving devices in the good old U.S. of A.

We can even look back to historical biblical times and imagine how physically active their lives must have been without a Stairmaster. Christ, the ultimate role model in everything pertaining to life, was a carpenter, which is a physically challenging, muscle-utilizing job. Without Black and Decker power tools He probably chopped down trees, hauled and carried logs, and "lifted" and "lowered" using a hammer instead of a dumbbell on a daily basis. Many of the disciples of Jesus fished for a living, with the white-collar IRS worker, Matthew, being an exception. Not only did they walk extraordinary distances, they swam, rowed the boat, and pulled in heavy loads of fish. How much do you think 153 large fish weighed on that day when Simon Peter had such a miraculous catch? "Weight training" was a natural part of their everyday life.

Au contraire, based on our modern lifestyles that offer more convenience and less necessary physical activity, weight training and cardiovascular exercise needs to be intentional and inculcated into our weekly lives.

Weight Training Comes in Many Different Shapes and Sizes

I can guess what you might be thinking: *You mean I have to weight train in addition to cardiovascular exercise?* Just hold onto your barbell because I have some good news. Weight training is just one of several activities, classified as anaerobic that will help you kiss flab goodbye. If you want to transform your body into a fit and strong one, any form of anaerobic exercise can help get you there. These activities differ from aerobic activities in that they are primarily carried out using stored energy or glycogen as opposed to an oxygen pathway (delivering glucose to the muscles from the bloodstream through breathing). Before you go getting bored, let me explain that you can sprint, jump, or throw something heavy (yea!) to produce anaerobic training effects. There's more good news: You carry these activities out for a short duration and then take a little rest. The goal of this type of exercise is developing muscles. Short bursts of exertion followed by periods of rest promote muscle building.

Strength usually peaks in our 20s and then begins a slow descent. As we age, we lose muscle, which means we require less and less calories. Usually we don't make the adjustment in our food intake to compensate for the muscle loss, which translates to pounds gained. I can safely assume that you would rather lose fat and keep your muscle, which is where resistance training comes in.

Resistance training, strength training, and weight lifting build and preserve lean muscle mass. Resistance training and strength training are interchangeable terms, while weight training is specific to lifting weights. Remember, the goal and advantage of all three is the same when it comes to weight loss: improving our muscle to fat ratio, which translates to an increase in our metabolic rate (burn, baby, burn). Popeye wasn't just strong from eating his spinach (though I will highly suggest that in chapter 8) but from squeezing the can so hard that it popped open. And he could consume a lot of spinach because he had the muscle to burn it up.

Just like cardio, resistance training works on behalf of your metabolism, and your health, as opposed to dieting which works against your metabolism and oftentimes your health. Remember, it's something you do instead of do without.

The Many Benefits of Weight Training

Let's review the weight loss benefits of resistance training. The biggie is an increase in lean muscle mass leading to a higher rate of energy burned which translates into an improved metabolism. Other important benefits to consider include helping prevent osteoporosis and improving the symmetry, posture, and therefore the appearance of our body. Osteoporosis, an age-associated condition of decreased bone density plays a responsible role in up to a million fractures annually in the United States. Bone density increases until about age 30, and then it begins to decrease. Regular exercise such as aerobic exercise and weight lifting inhibits the risk of osteoporosis, whereas dieting can actually perpetuate osteoporosis through limiting bone-building vitamins and minerals such as calcium and magnesium. One of the food groups often restricted in an attempt to decrease fat intake on many diets is dairy products. Although calcium can be obtained through nondairy sources such as beans, leafy greens, and nuts, some of the richest natural calcium sources are from dairy. But don't forget, these bone-building nutrients and food complexes have limited benefits without the weight bearing activity.[3]

Muscles and bones work in combination to hold your skeleton upright. This goes against gravity and therefore is a form of bearing weight. Additional movement, such as "lifting," stimulates bone formation and that is very good news, friends. Weight training is a promising tool for keeping your bones strong and healthy and fighting the aging process!

It Helps You Look Younger

For the icing on the cake, improving our muscularity is not only functional and practical for weight loss but it translates to a better and more youthful-looking body. Let's be honest, we all want to look good. Remember, we should do the best we can with what we've got. I once did body-composition measurements for a company that I was employed by. I measured the body fat of about 50 women over the course of a few days. These women were a variety of sizes: overweight, underweight, and ideal weight. The interesting thing was that some of the women who didn't need to lose any weight lacked tone. Their skin was loose and dimpled and their bodies looked haggard. This is where resistance training divides the fit from the trim. I believe this applies to being too thin as well. A body with good muscle tone appears younger.

Several years ago, I paced behind a very athletic looking "girl" in the Race for the Cure, which is an organized 5K run to raise money for cancer research. I ended up passing her and got the surprise of my life. She was not the twenty-something her backside portrayed. I introduced myself when we were receiving our awards and found out she was a 50-year-old distance runner, who looked darn good from any angle. I was surprised again because, although she was lean, she didn't have that wasted look that some distance runners have. After an informal interview, I found out her age-defying secret. It was in the weight room.

Looking good doesn't have to be all about good genetics and good plastic (surgery or credit cards). Exercise, especially the strengthening kind, allows us to dip into the fountain of youth energy and appearance wise. That's great news for our youth obsessed culture. Weakness and middle-age spread, associated with aging, are primarily results of inactivity. Strength training can turn back the biological clock.

It Helps You Live Longer

There's more good news about aging since it is something we are all doing ("outwardly we are wasting away").[4] Improvement in bone density, balance, and muscle strength can occur at any age. Some studies involving senior adults aged 70 and older revealed "astonishing" results after putting them through supervised exercise programs involving weight lifting, swimming, and stretching. Some of the seniors became stronger than their twenty-something attendants. Exercise, the strengthening kind, impacts quality of life and longevity.[5]

Basically, there are two major kinds of resistance training: isotonic and isometric and you're asking isowhat? Again this is good news because it broadens your options. Isotonic is a form of movement with resistance such as weight lifting, and isometric is resistance without movement such as a Pilates position that you hold. The choices are plentiful which means you are bound to find something you enjoy.

One of my clients once asked how I manage to make every training session totally different. That's one of the fun things about this kind of training. Resistance exercises, techniques, and equipment can be utilized and incorporated so that no two workouts are the same. For example, the core class that I teach involves Pilates, as well as the use of many different resistance toys to boost strength. Pilates poses, medicine balls, resistance balls, dumbbells, body bars, resistance bands, and BOSU balls can be utilized to improve strength, as well as balance and agility.

Everyone enjoys change and success can be related to methods matching your personality. You can also steal from tai chi and yoga to incorporate resistance into poses and movement. Even if we stick to one method such as weight training, there are numerous variations for each major muscle group. Speaking of which, since symmetry is an objective, the idea is to work all of the major muscles of the upper and lower body. The large muscles of the lower body include: quadriceps, hamstrings, gluteals, and calves. And the large muscles of the upper body include: chest, back, shoulders, biceps, triceps, and let's not forget our middle, the rectus abdominis.

How to Train Your Different Muscle Groups

When weight training, I try to follow an order so that I don't leave anything out. In general, the suggested progression is from large muscles to the smaller ones, performing at least one exercise per muscle group. If you have a weakness in certain muscles, those can be strengthened by adding more variations, more sets, more repetitions, or progressively heavier weight specific to that muscle. For example, many women have small, weak shoulders and might want to perform two exercises for the deltoids or shoulder muscles.

When utilizing other methods, such as Pilates, compound exercises in which more than one muscle group is emphasized, are common and time efficient. Currently, one of my favorite ways to train simply utilizes one's own body weight. Body resistance training has been popular for years because it is low maintenance. Like walking and running this requires no equipment and can be done anywhere, any time. Lunges, push-ups, and crunches are some quintessential examples of compound body resistance exercises. In fact, I tell everyone who uses time as their excuse for not strengthening their muscles that lunges, push-ups, and a couple of variations of basic crunches happen to work the quadriceps, the hamstrings, the calves, the gluteus muscles, the chest, triceps, shoulders, rectus abdominis, oblique muscles, and the back. In a time crunch, these few exercises are conveniently efficient.

Another related excuse for women is that they don't have time to change clothes. One solution might be to exercise in your stylish pumps, but let's get practical! My suggestion is to invest in some cute and comfortable double-duty clothes. If you have a corporate job with a strict dress code, this may not work for you. However, if your lifestyle allows for casual dressing and you are committed to making weight training happen, you don't have to look like a sweat hog. Hallelujah for velour!

Amy, a client I have trained on and off for eight years, loves the Kardio but dreads the weight room. She has lost 20 pounds and doesn't need to lose any more weight but rather wants to stay fit and strong for her children and her active husband. We alternate bouts of running and walking and in order to make it fun, I intermittently add body resistance exercises throughout the session. Without mandating weights, she is developing muscular strength and endurance.

I also think it's important to cater to your mood some days. If you're having a hard day, lighten up on yourself and do the bare minimum. Take the weight, sets, or reps down a notch. Remember, legalism usually catalyzes rebellion. In plain-speak, if you push yourself too hard consistently, you will associate pain with working out, joining the exercise dropouts of society. Remember, you are a lifer!

There are so many options to play with. You may find one thing and stick with it because you enjoy it. I have some advice if you are new to this type of training.

Take the One-Month Challenge

I am going to suggest that you try weight lifting for a few weeks. This conventional form of training the muscles will help educate and orient you toward musculoskeletal awareness. It's so helpful to learn the major muscle groups that need to be exercised regularly and to practice good form with slow and controlled movements. If you are a member of a health club, they usually offer at least one free consultation orienting the member to the equipment and offering a balanced regimen. If you avoid the gym scene, hire a good personal trainer for a few sessions and then pick up where you left off. If the budget is tight, consider hiring a trainer who will work with several people for an hour and recruit your friends to go in with you. Purchasing your own dumbbells and a weight-training book with pictures and descriptions of the exercises is helpful and can add time and freedom to your workout. Not to go unmentioned, there are a plethora of workout DVDs and cable-TV shows offering instruction.

The American College of Sports Medicine (ACSM) published researched guidelines for strength training for the general population. ACSM states that these should be viewed in context of the individual's target goals, physical capacity, and training status.

Resistance-training guidelines for healthy, sedentary individuals:

Exercise sequence:	large before small
Training frequency:	1-3 days per week
	8-12 repetitions maximum

I suggest starting at the lower end of these guidelines for the first week or two and then progress according to how your body is responding and how much you like the new activity. Since weight loss is a goal, stick with manageable weight per exercise. Lighter weight and more repetitions contribute more to leanness, whereas heavy lifting yields bigger muscles.

The bottom line is that a well-rounded weight-loss program includes aerobic exercise and strength training. (See chapter 12 for more specifics on Kardio and weight training)

~~~~~

I was giving the publishers of this book a tour of a weight-room facility when we bumped into a friend of mine we'll call "Don" because that's his name. Don is a guy who regularly works out with weights. After we introduced them to Don, we chatted and went on with our tour. My husband posed our friends the question, "How old do you think Don is?" They replied, "Oh, about 55, 56." My husband responded, "Actually Don is 81 years of age."

Don looks like he's in his mid 50s. That's without a tummy tuck, face lift, or bicep implant. Don's secret is consistent weight training coupled with Kardio—and of course faith in the Maker. I want to be like Don.

MAKE IT *happen*

I Can't **Weight** *to Get Started*

1. Remember that weight training is significantly helpful in the battle of the bulge.

2. Join a gym or purchase some weight appropriate dumbbells, a body resistance bar, or an exercise ball (the big ones).

3. Fast-forward to chapter 12 for more resistance training tips.

FAVORITE SMOOTHIE
Serves 2

1 cup frozen strawberries

¼ cup frozen raspberries

1 banana

juice of ½ lemon

1 cup apple juice

Put ingredients in the blender and blend until smooth.

I experiment with smoothies all the time, but this one is my daughter Nicole's favorite. If you aren't a big fruit eater, this is a good way to get your fruit servings in, and it can satisfy a craving for something sweet.

Strawberries are filled with phytonutrients. They are a rich source of phenols, which are potent antioxidants, making strawberries heart protective, anti-cancerous, and anti-inflammatory.

WILD BLUEBERRY SMOOTHIE
Serves 2

½ cup organic apple juice (apples have a high pesticide residue)

1 cup frozen wild blueberries (or cherries)

½ cup fresh diced pineapple

1 banana (fresh or frozen)

½ cup plain yogurt or kefir

Put all ingredients in the blender and blend until smooth. Wild blueberries are smaller than traditional ones and are packed at their peak.

I play with smoothie ingredients all the time so here are a couple of alternatives for 1 person (see next page).

WILD BLUEBERRY/CHERRY SMOOTHIE

Serves 1

½ cup milk (or soy milk or rice milk)

½ cup frozen wild blueberries

¼ cup frozen cherries

½ banana

Blueberries are an incredible source of antioxidant compounds as well as vitamin C and fiber.

TROPICAL SMOOTHIE

Serves 1

¾ cup frozen chopped pineapple

1 banana

2 tablespoons coconut nectar or low-fat coconut milk

½ cup low-fat plain yogurt

Combine ingredients in a blender until smooth.

This is a very satisfying smoothie and a delicious dessert option with the Super Food yogurt (see chapter 8).

Pineapple is rich in bromelain, which is made up of enzymes that aid digestion. Bromelain is also anti-inflammatory. Bananas are packed with potassium, which helps regulate heart function.

CHAPTER 7

EMBRACE RANDOM ACTS

**I buffet my body and
make it my slave.**

—*The apostle Paul*

M y first collegiate track meet was disastrous! My nerves took charge of my stomach and I was in the bathroom most of the hour before so I didn't get a proper warm-up. My coach was nowhere to be found. My warm-up was a quick 50-yard dash right before the race started. I had never raced the mile on an indoor track, so most of my focus went toward counting the number of times I had to go around (eight)...and I got lapped. The only exciting thing to tell is that I finished...finally.

In spite of a very rough start, I went on to compete in four more meets that same spring, finishing in the middle pack in every race. I was consistently confused about important details like when to "fall in" and where to finish. My lack of experience in competition was obvious to the other coaches, spectators, and competitors, I'm sure. Putting myself through the brutal intimidation of it all was not to keep a track scholarship, as you may have supposed. Instead, Eric Liddell's famous statement in *Chariots of Fire* resonates with me: "When I run, I feel His pleasure." Another huge motivation for me is the inherent joy in challenging my mind and body to comply and exert.

Did I mention that I was the only runner with two little girls on the sidelines yelling, "Go mommy, go!!" Basically, I was old enough to be the mother of my competitors at the time. (Non-collegiate athletes can compete in collegiate track meets as "unattached" runners.) I even went back to the 1500 on the track for more torture this year. I am a classic late bloomer and an "it's never too late" advocate—

- It's never too late to take up a sport you have always wanted to try.
- It's never too late to choose an active hobby.
- It's never too late to change the way you move throughout the day.

The apostle Paul loved to use athletic metaphors, especially about boxing and running, in the books he authored. In one of his spiritual analogies, he says that he buffets his body and makes his body his slave.[1] Our bodies should be like slaves in subjection to our minds and wills, instead of being the boss of us. So often we allow the body to dictate our choices, and the body is a poor leader. We must constantly decide what is best for our bodies and make them submit to our wills, even though it often goes against what feels good and what's culturally par for the course.

It's Time to Walk All Over the "Lazy System"

How does this relate to movement? It has vast ramifications. We must make a conscious effort to beat the system of convenience that is making us all fat and lazy. Modern conveniences are one of the things sabotaging our weight-loss efforts. We have eliminated so many opportunities for basic movement, and it's time to take them back. There are many simple ways to increase calorie burning, keep the metabolism stoked, and live an energetic and active life, all of which contribute to weight loss and help prevent weight gain as we age.

In the 1993 film *What's Eating Gilbert Grape?* Johnny Depp, as Gilbert, describes his 500-pound mother as "a beached whale." The severely obese Mrs. Grape hasn't left the house in over seven years. When she has to get up, the wood floors creak and almost cave in. She tragically tells Gilbert, "I never, never meant to be like this." She had become the poster lady for the couch potato who spends every waking, eating, and sleeping moment sitting or lying down.

Like Mrs. Grape, none of us plans to be overweight nor do we plan to be sedentary. It seems like everyday inactivity is promoted and activity is demoted, and sooner or later the statistics catch up to us. Have you noticed that physical activity has been progressively and subtly engineered out of our lives? We must intentionally and sometimes militantly take steps toward taking it back.

Step #1: Take Back Walking

One of the most obvious ways is to walk more. Incorporating more walking into our daily lives is probably not going to be the sole solution to our weight problem (refer back to chapter 5), but it is a baby step in the right direction. Take the stairs instead of the elevator or escalator, avoid the moving sidewalk at the airport, and save your money by giving up the valet parking at your favorite restaurants.

My husband and I went to a popular sushi restaurant the other night with parking right next to the door and plenty of spaces. The valet parkers were hoping to save us literally about 50 steps. JUST SAY NO...thank you. Instead of letting your dog set up land mines in the backyard or paying for the very chic dog-walking service, take him for a walk yourself (and bring your scooper). Your momentum may be stifled when Fido stops to smell all those cryptic messages left by his canine compatriots, but its okay, because you are getting off the couch! It may be the most exciting thing in your dog's day, and it's even more exciting that you are taking steps toward changing the way you move.

When you go to the mall, park your car as far from the entry as possible (in daylight) and power walk to your destination. Whenever possible make your walking powerful by using large arm movements and a brisk pace. Walking is the most basic human form of travel, and yet we do so little of it. Thomas Jefferson said, "Walking is the best possible exercise. Habituate yourself to walk very far."

In order for walking to be the best exercise, we would indeed have to walk very far or very fast. Remember intensity matters. But walking is the most accessible exercise. Walking more is a component of a total lifestyle overhaul that helps us get and stay lean. We have already discussed the obstacles to walking everywhere for most of us, citing the development of cities based on automobile transportation as one of the main deterrents, but that doesn't mean there aren't plenty of ambulatory opportunities.

Most would argue that another major inhibition to walking is saving time. However, we have eliminated walking from our lives even where no time is saved. Take the moving sidewalk in the airports, for example; you can power walk right past your travel buddies who opted for a ride, or if you're really in a hurry, power walk the moving sidewalk (stay left!).

Step #2: Take Back the Television (No, Really—to the Store)

Evaluate the deterrents to walking. Think about things that have sabotaged your walking. Swap some sedentary time with walking time. Quit watching the shopping channel; in fact, quit watching the tube in general, and move those limbs. Turning off the television is a calorie-burning hint worth implementing. The mere act of turning it off only burns a few calories at best, but the ramifications could burn thousands of calories over time and add life to your years! Women who watch between 20 and 40 hours of television weekly have a 68 percent higher risk of obesity, and as you could guess, TV viewing is significantly affiliated with adolescent obesity as well.[2]

If you must watch some TV, think outside the box and try doing housework during the commercials or doing crunches while you wait to see who's getting booted off your favorite unreality show. I haven't sat through a commercial in about 11 years (since the birth of my first daughter), instead, I do a quick chore. If you have a treadmill or stationary bike at home, combining Kardio with your must-watch show is a no brainer (especially considering most shows are 30 minutes—perfect!). Go against the sedentary flow and start becoming an active person. You would be surprised at how this spills over into every area of our lives. It's contagious!

Step #3: Take Back the Household Chores

Now think about all the ways modern conveniences have stolen our potential for burning calories in the kitchen, yard, and garage (burly men). Take it back not only for walking, but for any moving that has been delegated to devices. Cooking, cleaning, sewing, remodeling, yard work, car washing, and grocery shopping can add to the better half of the weight-loss solution (the something you do instead of do without). Some of these areas are more practical to adopt a do-it-yourself policy than others and some are more time intensive than others. Consider that we have delegated everything except sitting, and as a result, our clothes are no longer fitting.

I remember my mom telling me that anyone who can read can cook, and I have to agree. Instead of fast food or a frozen macaroni and cheese dinner, try grocery shopping and cooking. Mix it up in the kitchen instead of relying on boxed, frozen, canned, pre-packaged convenience foods, loaded with suspicious ingredients. I often forego food processors, mixers with a stand (I've yet to succumb to this supposed convenience), and electric juicers and use my hands to stir and chop. This category has huge ramifications. Not only are you burning calories by doing your own cooking, you will appreciate the food more. And an added benefit is that you are controlling what you put into your mouth as well as the mouths of those you love. Ingredients can benefit our health and metabolism or make us sick and tired, cranky, and overweight. Let's give our families the ingredients that will make a difference in their livelihood.

BECOME A DO-IT-YOURSELFER

If you adopt some of these ideas, let them include cooking and walking. I have become a "do it yourselfer" in the kitchen, and it saves my family untold calories, especially unnecessary sugar and unhealthy fat! My husband, my daughters, and my dog, who loiters in the kitchen when I'm cooking, absolutely love the fact that in the last several years I have been learning to make it myself. I'm not talking gourmet cooking but very simple, healthy food preparation.

I used to buy lemonade in a carton and now we use an inexpensive hand juicer. My seven-year-old usually makes the lemonade and homemade orange juice too. We used to rely on frozen organic waffles, not a bad choice, but now I like to make them with my idiot-proof, perfect every time, waffle maker. We don't have them every week but why should we have to leave our house to get waffles? Besides, I never met a recipe I didn't change for the health of it. When I made Belgian waffles for the first time, it was risky business. I substituted wheat flour for white, olive oil for most of the butter, eliminated the sugar (they use maple syrup on them, for goodness' sake), and used 2 percent milk instead of whole. I had low expectations. They turned out fabulous!!

I have a friend who is a "do it yourselfer" too, and she brought ingredients for ice cream to a birthday party one day, and we made our own baggy of ice cream without an ice cream maker (see recipe). Not only was it delicious, it was a blast, and you burn some calories shaking it for 20 minutes! I finally broke down and purchased an awesome ice-cream maker. You would not believe the difference between homemade and store-bought frozen yogurt, sorbets, ices such as green tea ice (see recipe), and ice cream. It is tasty fun for special occasions and saves you calories and artificial ingredients.

I hear gardening can be therapeutic and addictive. I'm not prone to gardening, but I appreciate the manicured yard of my next-door neighbor, and I can only imagine that he derived tremendous pleasure from his toil. You could save your Andrew Jackson and resist the temptation to buy that shiny automatic lawn mower or pay for mowing services and "do it yourself" with a push mower.

Robot vacuum cleaners, dry cleaners, car washes, and other hired-out or mechanized ways of getting chores done simply steal fat burning possibilities. I am a laundry freak. (Ben, my husband, says it would make my day if he would go out and collect dirty clothes from our neighbors just so I could wash them—not!) I am peevishly particular about laundry. Rarely do I let anyone else wash the clothes. Truth be told, it's not about the opportunity to sweat, but it is about sweaty clothes sitting in a hamper!

And speaking of shopping: the catalog, e-Bay, and the shopping channel may be costing you more than money. They could be costing you valuable calorie-burning opportunities.

Step #4: Take Back Playtime

Why do we think we are too old or too mature to play? Irish dramatist George Bernard Shaw said, "We don't stop playing because we grow old, we grow old because we stop playing." There are other ways to add to the calorie-burning equation apart from conventional exercises and lifestyle activity, and playing more qualifies.

If you are the parent of a young child, instead of paying a nanny or babysitter to play with your kids, get in touch with your outer child and play in the yard or a park. Until my oldest turned ten it was a weekly custom to go to the playground. We live in a climate where you can be outdoors at least part of the day about 360 days a year (in Texas they say if you don't like the weather, just wait a minute). Our family not only enjoys the outdoorsy activities, but we might go stir-crazy if we couldn't be outside. We've factored in more playing, which is one way of making an active lifestyle a family affair.

One day I went to the playground with a friend and her kids, and she commented: "No wonder you stay so fit, I'm tired just watching you." I was on the monkey bars, the slide, and the bouncy horse with the kids before I finally collapsed on the bench next to her to visit.

Some of my favorite experiences with my children are related to playing. What started out as an attempt to connect on their level, became a childlike freedom for me to play. I am transported to the memories and wonder of carefree moments in time. The awe and wonder of this God-breathed intricately functioning body that can go from standing to running with a signal from brain to body or sitting to jumping at will and command, is still truly amazing. We jump on the trampoline weekly (except when it's 100 degrees). We wrestle and play running games around the house, and one of our favorite things to do is to crank up the music and dance (yes, some Baptists dance). We walk our beloved retriever most days, and we chase her plenty because she is an escape artist like all pets.

It doesn't take a rocket scientist to figure out that if the parents are active, the kids are more likely to be active; and if your spouse is active, you are much more likely to be active; and if your friends are active…and so on.

It doesn't matter how or what you like to play, playing burns calories. Whether you have your own children, grandchildren, nieces, nephews… all kids love to play. When you are active, energetic, and fit, the kids around you will love it and will follow your lead.

I'm not the first chosen for Pictionary—I lack the drawing gene—but my daughter realized in pre-K that I am a good pick for tag. We didn't outgrow these games; we became thinkers instead of players! Unfortunately kids are following suit and growing out of physical play by the time they are in junior high. They trade in their Nikes for Game Boys and their ballet shoes for Play Stations. The average child only burns a mere 100 calories per hour of sedentary video playing.

Get your kids to help you with the yard work instead. They could burn up to 600 calories an hour. Also, try replacing their handhelds with the new physically interactive games like the ones with the mini–dance floors or interactive golf. These are a blast, and they will get your kids moving more.

Step #5: Take Back the Active Vacation

Another take on play is planning active vacations. So many times we see vacations as a time to sit around. Instead, take a vacation from sitting (what we do most days) and get moving with trips that center around a sport or activity such as snow skiing, biking, hiking, camping, rock climbing, rafting, and touring, or make a point to incorporate activity into vacations.

I have a client who just returned from sightseeing in London. We had worked hard to get her into a weight-loss pattern, so I gave her a "just maintain" speech and the bit about "all things in moderation" (the English aren't known for eating healthfully or moderately, think scones and creamy, sugary tea). She was stupefied to discover a five-pound weight loss upon return. Movement can go a long way—they walked a lot!

If you like beach vacations, swim in the ocean. If you like the mountains, climb a fourteener with your friends. Community service or mission ventures are philanthropic and are often awesome opportunities for moving as well, full of serving, building, and laboring as opposed to sitting, eating, and fiddling. We have a retired friend who gets joy and exercise by helping with Habitat for Humanity yearly.

Just jump on the Internet and check out the wide variety of active vacations that are offered. They have affordable or luxurious options for singles, couples, or families who want to soak in the beauty as well as keep their hearts pumping.

Step #6: Take Up a New Sport

Another extensive area where we could significantly increase our caloric expenditure is through sports…no, not watching them. It's never too late to take up _____ (fill in the blank with that sport you've always wanted to try). My husband is teaching all of us to surf, and we both picked up wakeboarding a few years ago. He is passionate about surfing. I prefer wakeboarding, but I admit surfing is more practical since we don't have a boat but we do live near the ocean. Although a spa day is a great getaway, consider asking for a more activity-inspiring gift for your next birthday. For instance, my husband sent me off to wakeboarding camp, and I came home completely energized.

Instead of the book club or the needlepoint group—adding more sedentary hours to the week—join the croquet club or the racquetball league. You're never too out of shape to join a walking club. Get fit and social by joining any number of leagues (tennis, soccer, swimming) for adults. I trained a single 30-something who was in an adult co-ed tennis league. She's married now. You never know! The YMCA, community centers, or your local church are good bets for finding adult sport opportunities.

Enter a local 5K, and if you don't train to jog or run it, power walk it. Many average people—not super-fit types—take on a big challenge like the marathon or a sprint triathlon (sounds scary, but it is actually a short version of a triathlon) just to increase their commitment to fitness and exercise. A 5K is much more doable, in my opinion, and training for it is an excellent way to lose weight. K, in this case, stands for kilometers, and 5 is the number of kilometers, which is equal to the 5000 meters that you will cover in the event. If you still have no idea what that means, I'm not alone. I think in plain, American miles, so a 5K is 3.1 miles, or 12 ½ times around the school track. The standard community-sponsored "fun" run, also called a run/walk, is a 5K, which means it is long enough that you will want to be prepared, even if you are planning to power walk it. A 5K can start you on your way to getting fit and shedding pounds. Additionally, a training focus rewards you with a sense of accomplishment for trying something new.

Most walkers and runners sign up for this race just for the fun of it. So don't worry about competing for the blue ribbon, or being intimidated. I have run in plenty of 5Ks and you see all types. Before you register for the next 5K in your area, call your local YMCA, look in the newspaper or local health and fitness periodicals, or check out www.runnersworld. com for good training programs. The registration fee is usually nominal, and you get a T-shirt for your hard earned francs.

A good goal if you are a first-timer is to just go the distance and have fun doing it. Preparation for the race is more about maximizing weight loss and getting excited about your long-term journey to fit and lean.

Speaking of long-term journeys, one man named Steve had a lot of weight to lose, so he set out on an adventure…a trek across America. Steve trekked through 15 pairs of shoes, 6 backpacks, and over 30 pairs of socks on his roughly 3000-mile hike from California to Manhattan, losing 100 pounds in the process. Steve said of his experience, "This is not about obsessing about numbers, or times, or dates, or miles. It's just about going on a walk and sort of having time to get things straight." He didn't measure the food he ate or use a pedometer, and he said one of his aims was behavior change. It sounds like we share the same aversion to focusing on the small picture. The guy simply and determinedly walked his way/weight leaner. A lot of small steps added up to some huge emotional, mental, and life-changing steps for Steve. A bystander who witnessed the completion of the journey said, "I think it's great that he's finished his goal. So few of us actually keep them."

What a refreshing comment, considering he weighed in at 410 pounds at the start of his journey. This woman is praising him for keeping a non-weight related goal. He may be nowhere near his ideal weight, but it was more about the journey, the experience, the emotional health benefits of movement, being outdoors, and trying something new and risky. The inescapable benefit was weight loss.[3]

This is an extreme example, but any of us can take on a new movement challenge and reap so much more than weight loss. The intangibles of setting out to do something like learn a new sport or complete a 400-yard swim are significant in keeping us motivated.

The Real Skinny on Movement

Bottom line, our food intake has not been modified to make up for our highly mechanized, sedentary lifestyle. And though our fat intake has declined slightly in the last few years, the quality of our food consumption in nutrition and freshness has dramatically declined, negatively affecting our waistlines. Boost your weight-loss potential by taking movement back (and take fresh food back while you're at it—chapter 8).

I'll tell you what…if you will try something new, I will too. I have always wanted to do a triathlon, but I'm not very good at swimming. The excuse clauses can hold us back from ever setting goals or dreaming dreams. Let's show the excuses what we're made of!

In the hilarious movie *What about Bob?*, Bob (Bill Murray) is a multiphobic neurotic. He is encouraged by his new therapist, Dr. Leo Marvin (Richard Dreyfus), to take *Baby Steps*—the title of Dr. Marvin's new book—toward mental health (curing his phobias). Bob excitedly takes baby steps around the room, showing insane enthusiasm for the new program. He says, "All I have to do is take one little step at a time, and I can do anything." I'm encouraging you to take baby steps toward a very active way of life. (*Baby Steps to a Lean Way of Life* was a potential title for this book.) These are some ideas for reincorporating opportunities for movement back into your life. But remember your personality and preferences will come into play. Make it fun!

MAKE IT
happen

"Take It Back" Moves

1. Instead of riding, take the stairs.

2. Get cooking.

3. Garden (weeding, planting, hoeing).

4. Push the lawn mower.

5. Clean house (vacuum, sweep, scrub)

6. Make TV time exercise time (or at least do both at the same time).

7. Park inconveniently (the far side of the parking lot).

8. Shop 'til you drop (no wallet necessary).

9. Walk or bike instead of driving, when possible.

10. At the office—get up and move every chance you get or use your chair as an exercise prop.

11. Wash windows.

12. Chop wood.

13. Paint the house.

14. Help out with physical labor through community or mission service.

Calories burned per hour of activity

Activity (1 hour)	Calories burned based on body weight[4]		
	130 lbs	155 lbs	190 lbs
Basketball	354	422	518
Bowling	177	211	259
Cleaning, heavy, vigorous effort	266	317	388

Cleaning, house, general	207	246	302
Cooking or food preparation	148	176	216
Croquet	148	176	216
Dancing, general	266	317	388
Gardening, general	295	352	431
Golf, general	236	281	345
Horseback riding, general	236	281	345
Horseback riding, trotting	384	457	561
Moving furniture, household	354	422	518
Mowing lawn, general	325	387	474
Painting, papering, plastering, scraping	266	317	388
Pushing or pulling stroller with child	148	176	216
Scrubbing floors, on hands and knees	325	387	474
Skiing, water	354	422	518
Soccer, casual, general	413	493	604
Surfing, body or board	177	211	259
Sweeping garage, sidewalk	236	281	345
Table tennis, Ping-Pong	236	281	345
Tennis, general	413	493	604
Volleyball, beach	472	563	690
Walk/run-playing with child(ren)	236	281	345

DO-IT-YOURSELF ICE CREAM

Burn a few calories with this indulgence

This is super fun for kids parties and does not require an ice-cream maker. It is messy (ice melts), so I recommend making it an outside or poolside gig. You will need:

gallon-size zip-lock bags

sandwich-size zip-lock bags

sugar

milk

vanilla

spoons

Put 1 tablespoon sugar, ½ cup of milk (or ½ and ½), and ¼ teaspoon of vanilla in a sandwich bag and seal completely. Put 2 tablespoons of rock salt (find on baking aisle) in a gallon-size bag. Put the filled sandwich bag and ice to fill the large bag ¾ full. Shake and roll filled bag over and over until frozen (about 18 minutes). Ta-da! Eat from the bag delicious homemade ice cream.

GREEN-TEA SHAVED ICE

A nice summer treat for an adult party—makes approximately 2½ quarts

A nice summer treat for an adult party

6 cups water

1 cup honey

2 teaspoons grated orange peel

8 green (or black) tea bags

½ cup lemon juice

limes to garnish bowls (optional)

Combine water, honey, and orange peel in a large saucepan. Bring to a boil over medium heat and then remove from heat. Place tea bags in the pan and steep for about 10 minutes. Remove the bags and cool to room temp. Stir in juice and pour into an ice-cream canister. Freeze in the ice-cream maker (according to directions). You could also pour the cooled concoction into a glass baking dish and freeze in your freezer if you don't have an ice-cream maker.

CHAPTER 8

EMBRACE FOOD

**Food is our common ground,
a universal experience.**

—James Beard

One Christmas holiday, I was away from home. I can remember having trouble falling asleep and feeling a yearning for comfort. Finding a book in the room where I was staying, I turned to the Psalms. It wasn't the first time that I had read the Bible, but somehow this time it seemed to apply to me more directly and in a way I hadn't known before. Perhaps it was because I was in those critical teenage years, when you really begin to own your identity. What I found was that God was revealing Himself to me personally. He had already been using circumstances, friends, and exposure to church to woo me—prior to this, some acquaintances had invited me to Fellowship of Christian Athletes functions, but I didn't want to make time in my schedule to fraternize with the God squad, so I had politely declined. I suspect those same people were praying that I would recognize my need for God. On that quiet, holiday night, I did, and He met me there.

This was a defining time for me—when I accepted the truth that God is both good and in control of everything and that this truth has direct implications for how I should live my life. I started going to those FCA meetings I had turned down before and made a commitment to read the Bible every day for the next year (which I did). Within months I was selected to be the female president of FCA for the following year, and I was going full speed ahead in my spiritual journey. I dove headfirst into Christianity, driving myself to a nondenominational church in my little orange Fiat (how I wish I still had that car), going to group Bible studies, sharing my faith in God with others on the street, late-night prayer meetings, memorizing Scripture, tithing, fasting, and, in my commitment to sexual purity, even vowing to stop kissing my boyfriend (he was less than thrilled). Some called me a "Jesus Freak"; others gave it a more positive spin, saying I was "on fire for God." The truth is, I was incredibly blessed to be given the opportunity to hear God's Word shared through gifted speakers and musicians (Christian music was exploding onto the scene in the early '80s). I had been changed and was sincerely into pursuing this new way of life.

The Perfect Storm

My spiritual conversion had a ripple effect in my life and effectively transformed me in many areas. I had not, however, experienced its impact on my physical being. More specifically, it had not really changed how I felt *about* my body or how I felt *in* my body. All I knew at that time was that I didn't feel *good.*

There were so many factors in the crowded equation of my growing up season. For instance, every one of my girlfriends beat me to "the change." By the time I finally came around, my girlfriends weren't discussing such things in detail, nor did I feel comfortable talking about it—I suppose you don't discuss what you don't completely understand. So I was unprepared for such an abrupt change, both externally and internally. I wasn't too hyped about the pounds this new womanly figure was giving me, and I was oblivious to the impact my hormones were having on my energy, emotions, and metabolism.

Adding havoc to the struggles I didn't know I was struggling with, my eating habits were atrocious and had been for years, with no visible consequences. I had no self-control in relation to food because I had never had to. Eating whatever I wanted usually meant fatty, sugary foods. One year some of the guys affectionately dubbed me "Cookie Monster" because I was more than happy to eat their cookies and any other sweets offered to me at lunch. One of my favorite hobbies besides cheerleading and tennis consisted of consuming large quantities of processed foods, which I now know added insult to my "not feeling good."

From Cookie Monster to Twiggy

Add "the change" and my eating habits together, and that equaled to the 15 pounds I gained that year. I quickly went tumbling from the top of the cheerleading pyramid to the very bottom. No matter what, I was going to be thin again, I determined. And so I was. My senior year, the football coaches called me "Twiggy" because my 90-pound frame resembled that of the extremely thin British model from the 60s. I was a "thin at all costs" poster child, and I didn't even recognize it.

Then the summer before my senior year came along…and it went. It was the strangest thing. I was at a high school friend's surprise birthday bash not too long ago, and that's where I discovered that I had no recollection of that summer. At the party, my friends were recounting all the fun and embarrassing memories. I laughed and reflected. But when I went to bed that night, I felt very disturbed. One of my close friends had shared a story about our time at FCA camp. FCA camp? I had forgotten that we all went to camp. Through the various puzzle pieces provided in their stories, I was able to come away with some surface facts about this seemingly lost event from my past. But I tried my best to retrieve an actual memory—getting there, the flag football game she had mentioned, where we stayed—and nothing came to me.

In retrospect, there was no wondering *why* I couldn't remember. I knew that full well, as I lay in bed and mourned the loss. That summer, I was so nutritionally bankrupt, I couldn't think straight. I wasn't taking in or digesting enough calories to keep my mind and body in good health. Restriction, depletion, and dehydration had left me strung out.

And so had the eating disorder that consumed so much time and energy during those years.

If I were to analyze it, which I didn't dare, I would have seen that I was disassociating my treatment of my body from my identity. It's a lot like our inability to see the connections between our habits and the circumstances we often bring on ourselves. Denial would be the appropriate word for this. I analyzed and studied many deeply spiritual matters during those spiritually formative years, but body philosophy, including *how should we then eat,* simply was not one of them.

Thinking About the Way We Think About Food

If I were to apply the old saying, "You are what you eat," to those whirling dervish years, sometimes I was "not much," and other times I was a good helping of "sugar and spice and everything processed." My weight was out of control because my eating was out of control. My eating was out of control because my way of thinking about food and the body was out of control. I had to change my way of thinking in order to make peace with food and with my body.

After examining body image in chapter 4, I hope you have started to rethink your own body philosophy in terms of scriptural implications. St. Paul said that no one ever hated his own body but nourishes and cherishes it,[1] and this applies not only to how we should view the body, but also to how we should feed the body in light of this view. Grasping this concept is as vital to having balance in our spiritual and personal lives as our views on politics or sex and sexuality.

Speaking of sex, we don't talk about it from God's viewpoint nearly as much as we should. Most of us aren't sure how we *actually* feel and how we *ought* to feel about sex and our sexuality. Sex is woven into the fabric of our beings by God Himself, and yet integrating sexuality with our faith seems to be asking too much of ourselves. In spite of our cultural conditioning, I'll bet I could get you to agree that kissing is much more than two lips coming together. So how could sex be merely two bodies coming together? How do we mesh our feelings about sex with our religious views?

The problem is, we usually don't. But what if we truly pondered sexuality through God's eyes, seeing it as holy and glorifying, as He does? Let me just say that it sheds a whole new light on and adds a fascinating dimension to our sex lives. In the same way, we don't tend to associate eating with holiness. Our food philosophy, or lack of one, hasn't bred the kind of congruency Paul is talking about. And this is made evident by our weight problems.

Interestingly, we could look at some of the same Scriptures to develop the proper sex philosophy *and* the proper food philosophy, killing two birds with one verse, so to speak. For example: "Present your body as a living and holy sacrifice, acceptable to God, which is your spiritual service of worship"; or "Do you not know that your body is a temple of the Holy Spirit, who is in you, whom you have received from God? You are not your own, you were bought with a price. Therefore, honor God with your body."[2] Both of these verses are about what we put into our bodies, as well as what we put our bodies into (applied to male sexuality). As God's children, we must bring every aspect of our bodies under His rule and authority.

The right philosophy is all about motives too. See, we can do the right things with the wrong motives. In other words, are our healthy eating practices motivated by the desire to measure up to societal standards of what looks good, or are we motivated by the desire to be good to our bodies because this is pleasing to God? By the same token, do we abstain from extramarital sex because we don't want to get pregnant or get an STD? Or is our motivation more about trusting that God knows what is best (and most pleasurable too) for us? If you answered *yes* to the first one in each case, how far do you think you can carry it? I would venture to say that the higher the purpose, the greater the follow-through and success rate.

What's Your Take on Food?

So now that we know the proper philosophies toward food and sexuality, let's get a little more personal and evaluate where we stand. It may seem bizarre to have a personal food philosophy, but trust me, we are acting one out daily, so we might as well get it out on the table. Some might say food is life or food is comfort or food is pleasure. Others might see food as the enemy. One thing I have observed, though it should come as no profundity, is that our personal food philosophy greatly impacts how we eat. Let's take a look at how a couple of different philosophies have affected others' eating habits.

The Fitness Industry's Take

Having been in the fitness business for several years, I have noticed that a lot of these people see food simply as a means to an end. It is mainly fuel for athletic efficiency and better appearance, and this could take one down a deviant path as you will recall (from chapter 4). A lot of my peers in the fitness industry, including the nutritionists, recommend things like protein powders and bars, NutraSweet, saccharine, Snackwell's cookies and crackers, fat-free butter (as if), and fat-free mayonnaise, as well as other fake foods as long as they produce a specific outcome. Never mind the process, literally. The emphasis is on no/low calorie, no/low fat, or no/low carbs, and this is all they're looking for on the nutrition label. Many are also pro pills and potions as means to an end. If carried to the nth degree, even steroids could be justified as useful fuel.

Most people assume that I would fall in this category because I'm admittedly a workout nut. But the telling difference would be the word "diet" before most of their foods. In contrast to them, I steer clear of anything with the word "diet" in it. Truth be told, many of these "fitness gurus" are diet advocates, without regard to the healthfulness, or lack thereof, of the foods they and their eager clients are actually consuming. But all you have to do is look around to see that exercise alone won't make a body fit or healthy.

The Whole-Food Industry's Take

At the other end of the food spectrum is the whole-foods or natural-foods movement. These food "purists" are particular about animal rights, hugging trees, recycling, being kind to the soil, and farming standards and procedures: for example, organic, farm-raised, cage-free or free-range, hormone-free and they pay attention to the ingredients.

However, they might not be interested in limiting their intake of "healthy" but calorie-dense and super-fatty foods, and some in this camp would justify packaged foods like toaster tarts, frozen waffles, boxed macaroni and cheese, and cheese puffs because the word "organic" or "natural" is slapped across the label.

There's Truth in There Somewhere

We can learn from these groups and their eating habits. In fact, we could take some ideas from both, weed out some of the faults of both, add on, elaborate and tweak, and come up with a solid eating philosophy that could help us improve our health, and reach our ideal weight and keep us there. That's where I have landed in the last 15 years—trying to merge a lean-eating philosophy with a wholesome, natural food philosophy, and I have nothing extra to show for it.

Weight control, in my opinion, is about balancing eating for pleasure and eating for health, because they are intrinsically woven. If we leave out one of these components, which many diets do, it can lead to imbalance in our lives and could manifest itself physically. For example, if we eat for fuel and leave out pleasure, we miss out on the delight of food, possibly leading to underweight or asceticism or finally giving in and bingeing. On the other hand, eating for pleasure *only* puts us on the path to gluttony and being chronically overweight and paves the way for indulgence across the proverbial life board.

The truth is, food touches just about every aspect of life. It helps us grow, thrive, and heal throughout life. Food also plays a big part in social interactions, connecting us to those around us. We also can be emotionally nurtured, as in we feel secure and provided for, when our bodies are nurtured. Tastes and smells bring back memories of wonderful events in our lives. In essence, food is a great gift from the Source of all gifts. But when we take the gift for granted, it can become the source of immense pain. So what does the Source think about food?

God's Take on Food

God gave us food for sustenance as well as for pleasure: "I give you every seed-bearing plant on the face of the whole earth and every tree that has fruit with seed in it. They will be yours for food....God saw all that He had made, and it was very good."[3]

It is foundational to understand that food keeps us alive. When the Israelites were leaving Egypt, God provided manna, which was not beautiful nor desirable but sustaining. Their journey from Egypt involved humbling them with manna in order to prepare them for the milk and honey of the Promised Land. This symbolizes the difference between mere sustenance and bountiful pleasure.

Later on, in the Psalms, King David rejoices in the pleasure aspect: "He makes grass grow for the cattle, and plants for man to cultivate— bringing forth food from the earth: wine that gladdens the heart of man, oil to make his face shine, and bread that sustains his heart."[4] Now we're talking, food is not just fuel, but it affects us emotionally too: "wine that *gladdens*…and bread that sustains *the heart.*"

The fact that God made so many varieties of plants, herbs, fruits, and vegetables, many brightly colored and some beautiful like the piece of fruit that Eve saw as pleasing to the eye and desirable, attests to His creating food for pleasure as well. God made food pleasing, satisfying, luscious, and rich as we know from having eaten things like a juicy pear or a ripe avocado or from drinking goat's milk and eating cheese and…after all, God gave us the essentials for creating such rich dishes as fettuccine alfredo and such delicious desserts as tiramisú and bread pudding. Food engages almost all of our senses: sight, touch, taste, and smell, delighting us on multiple levels.

Food and biblical history go hand in hand. Our recorded biblical history starts and ends with food playing a major symbolic and "sin"bolic role. Interestingly, the Bible reveals that food can be at the center of temptation, miraculous provision, or thanksgiving. Of course, the temptation started in the Garden of Eden, continued with Esau trading his birthright for stew, Daniel refusing the king's rich fare for more modest vegetables, and the temptation of Christ when He refused to turn stones into bread, in spite of incredible hunger.

The miracles involving food are many, including manna from heaven, God's miraculous provision for Elijah and the widow from Zarephath, and Christ "feeding the five thousand and gving thanks to God in front of them all." The thanksgiving for food is best evidenced in the last supper, when Christ took the bread, broke it, and gave thanks, and then again when Christ appears to two of the disciples on the road to Emmaus,

He finds Himself at the table with them. He again gave thanks before breaking the bread and partaking. Paul continued this tradition, giving thanks for the meal connecting heaven and earth, acknowledging the source of provision.[5]

From the fruit in Genesis to the feast in Revelation, food serves as the bookends of the Bible. Sadly, the tremendous spiritual symbolism of food and feasting is hardly ever talked about amongst God's people in the church. Eating involved more than sustaining the body in biblical times. It was steeped in sanctity. Think about Mount Sinai when Moses and the elders ate together, making their covenant with God official. Jacob and his father-in-law, Laban, sealed their pact through partaking of a meal together. When food was not available in Canaan, Joseph was reunited with his brothers through the provision of food. Jesus turned water to wine at a wedding celebration, symbolizing God's ability to make the ordinary extraordinary.[6]

And let's look more closely at that last supper mentioned briefly above. This most symbolic meal has had lasting meaning, as we still take the elements in remembrance of Christ.[7] God chose to use something we put in the body to symbolize His indwelling presence. The bread and the wine in their bareness remind us that He provides enough and He Himself is enough. Do we see the bread as holy, or have we, in our abundance, become so desensitized that we simply see the bread as stale?

We can glean much from the food references and symbolism in the Bible. In fact, it is a piece of the weight-loss puzzle. Food symbolizes God's provision and is something worth giving thanks for, celebrating, and sharing. Through understanding some things about the biblical history of food, which far exceeds the culinary, we can link our spiritual lives to our physical lives. This helps heal a distorted take on food.

One of the Best Gifts of the Earth: Food

As I was doing my research for this chapter, a beautiful passage surfaced. Reading it serves as a review for the things we have contemplated:

> The LORD your God is bringing you into a good land—a land with streams and pools of water, with springs flowing in the

valleys and hills; a land with wheat and barley, vines and fig trees, pomegranates, olive oil and honey; a land where bread will not be scarce and you will lack nothing; a land where the rocks are iron and you can dig copper out of the hills. When you have eaten and are satisfied, praise the LORD your God for the good land he has given you. Be careful that you do not forget the LORD your God, failing to observe his commands, his laws and his decrees that I am giving you this day. Otherwise, when you eat and are satisfied, when you build fine houses and settle down, and when your herds and flocks grow large and your silver and gold increase and all you have is multiplied, then your heart will become proud and you will forget the LORD your God, who brought you out of Egypt, out of the land of slavery. He led you through the vast and dreadful desert, that thirsty and waterless land, with its venomous snakes and scorpions. He brought you water out of hard rock. He gave you manna to eat in the desert, something your fathers had never known, to humble and to test you so that in the end it might go well with you. You may say to yourself, "My power and the strength of my hands have produced this wealth for me." But remember the LORD your God, for it is he who gives you the ability to produce wealth, and so confirms his covenant, which he swore to your forefathers, as it is today.[8]

Just look at all the beneficial foods listed in the above passage, also called the "seven species" of the land of Israel: wheat, barley, pomegranates, fig trees, olive oil, honey, bread (see biblically inspired soup below). The Bible can be an inspiration to the way we eat, the way we cook and do meals, and the way we diet or refuse to diet. God has provided food, and it is good. Let us rejoice and be glad in it. Let us eat and drink to the glory of God.

MAKE IT
happen

Let the Healing Begin By...

Giving thanks. For thousands of years in many traditional Jewish homes, when bread is "broken" and shared, they pray "Blessed are you O Lord our God, King of the universe, who brings forth bread from the earth." Acknowledging and thanking the Provider for His abundant provision is where we begin. If you would start each meal with a heart of gratitude for what is put before you, you will begin to experience freedom from fear, addiction, and bondage. I am talking specifically and practically of praying before and over meals. This is still a challenge for me.

After years of "saying grace," as it's known in the South, I still find myself going through the motions instead of truly pausing to be grateful. I still forego this simple act of gratitude too often in a rush to get to "what is necessary." I still sometimes expect to be satisfied completely by food, and I still struggle to understand that I do not live by bread alone but by God's allowing every breath I take.

Celebrating. One of the most common ways we celebrate together is by eating together. Think about it. Hardly a momentous occasion in life occurs without festivities centered around friends, family, and, of course, lots of food. Weddings, birthdays, and holidays are marked by memorable meals rooted in culinary traditions. Our get-togethers should constitute celebrating, not only centering around the consumption of the meal but in the opportunity to share memorable moments together.

I can identify with Abraham. When the three angelic visitors came to his home, he had everyone running around like chickens with their heads cut off to get food to them.[9] Instead of rushing to prepare meals and then hurrying through meals with family and friends, we must learn to savor the communal act of eating. I am trying to get my children involved in meal preparation and serving, so that we can share the burden and the joys of hosting.

Another aspect of celebrating mealtimes, which we rush past, is simply reclining at the table afterward. We are apt to go back to business as usual after we have filled our stomachs, when this could be prime fellowship time. I am so often guilty of waitressing and being anxious about getting the dirty dishes in the dishwasher.

Sharing is something that brings blessings to the people around us. In a day when anything homemade is hard to come by, the sharing of thoughtfully prepared food is such a delight. I learned this from a sweet friend from my youth who would "reach out" to others with a home-cooked or homemade gift. My mother-in-law, who is an incredibly thoughtful person, has also influenced me in this. When she makes soup, she loves to leave some on our doorstep (and often beautiful flowers too).

The joy that we get when we share food, whether it be through having friends into our home or through simply giving from the bountiful provision we possess, puts an equally joyous smile on the face of the receiver. Delivering a home-cooked meal to a friend who has been hospitalized or recently moved or who has a newborn baby is a welcome relief from the burden of meal prep or the practical, but not ideal, option of fast food. I get even more joy in knowing that what I am giving brings nourishment, energy, and nutrition to their table. See some easy to share, highly nutritious, and awfully delicious (I think) recipes below.

JACOB'S LENTIL SOUP

1 ½ cups split red lentils

6 cups chicken or vegetable stock

1 medium onion cubed

2 sticks chopped celery

1 carrot, cubed

1 leek, chopped

½ teaspoon ground cumin

1 tablespoon white wine vinegar

olive oil

salt

freshly ground black pepper

Put the lentils in a pot with the stock and vegetables and bring to a boil. Simmer for 30 minutes, until the lentils have disintegrated. If too thick, add water. Add cumin and wine vinegar and season to taste. Sauté the sliced onion in the olive oil until almost caramelized and add to the soup. Serve hot.[10]

Lentils are a wonderful source of cholesterol-lowering fiber, and they help stabilize blood sugar. They are also associated with a reduced risk of breast cancer. Leeks are a good source of vitamins C and B_6 and folic acid.

NUTTY GRANOLA
Makes enough to share

8 cups rolled oats

2 cups chopped almonds

1 cup chopped pecans

$1/3$ cup olive oil

$2/3$ cup honey

2 teaspoons vanilla

1 cup whole ground flaxseed meal

Preheat oven to 350°. Combine oats and nuts in a large bowl. Warm honey and oil on stovetop until they easily blend; do not boil. Add vanilla and whisk together. Pour over oat mixture and stir well. Spread mixture into two deep cookie sheets. Bake for 15 minutes and stir. Bake for another 15 minutes and stir. If necessary, bake for 5-7 minutes more until light golden brown. Do not cook to dark brown or the mixture will taste bitter. Remove from the oven and sprinkle the flaxseed over the mix. (If adding sesame seeds or chocolate, sprinkle those over the mixture too.) Stir thoroughly. Cool. Can be stored in jars or plastic containers for about ten days or can be frozen.

This recipe is one that I rarely make the same way twice. Substitute walnuts, cashews, peanuts, or pistachios for the pecans. You could add 1 cup of dark sesame seeds (after baking) for variety or ½ cup of dark chocolate pieces (just after baking) to make it an occasional treat or a decadent gift. You could make a citrus version by including orange or lemon zest. You can add dried fruit such as raisins, cranberries, or dates. You could use maple syrup instead of honey and so on and so on…Enjoy!

Flaxseed has a myriad of health benefits (anti-cancer, hormone balancing) and is a great source of fiber and the omega-3 healthy fats that so many of us are missing from our diets. Almonds also contain omega-3s.

SALMON WITH CORN AND ASPARAGUS
Serves 4

kernels of 2 ears of fresh, uncooked corn

1 bunch of asparagus or about 20 stalks, trimmed

1 anise fennel bulb or 2 small fennel bulbs, cut into ¼-inch wedges

a few sprigs from the fennel

1 onion cut into ¼-inch wedges

1 cup grape or cherry tomatoes, cut in half

8 cloves garlic

2 tablespoons olive oil

2 teaspoons balsamic vinegar

4 4-5 ounce wild salmon fillets

juice of one lemon

2 teaspoons of Provence Herbs (a mix of thyme, rosemary, and laurel found in specialty grocery stores—optional)

1 teaspoon of coarse salt

freshly ground pepper

Preheat oven to 400 degrees. Place corn kernels, asparagus, fennel bulbs and sprigs, onion, tomatoes, and garlic in a 10-by-15-inch baking dish. In a small bowl, whisk together olive oil and balsamic vinegar and drizzle over veggies. Place in the oven for twenty minutes. Wash the salmon and pat dry with a paper towel and place in the middle of the baking dish. Pour lemon juice over salmon and veggies and sprinkle ½ teaspoon of herbs on each salmon fillet (optional). Sprinkle salt and grind a bit of pepper over the mixture and return it to the oven. Bake for about 10 minutes (fish should flake). Peel the skin off or remove with a paring knife, place in the middle of each plate and surround with the veggies.

We eat salmon at least once a week. I absolutely love this recipe because it has so many unique and bold flavors. Your family and friends will think you labored in the kitchen for hours over this one dish meal.

Salmon is an amazing protein source boasting omega-3s, protein, potassium, selenium, and vitamin B_{12}.

Tomatoes are low calorie, nutrition powerhouses. They have vitamin C, carotenes (including lycopene), biotin, and vitamin K in abundance as well as a good amount of dietary fiber.

DOMENICA'S HERB-AND-NUT-CRUSTED HALIBUT
Serves 4

4 fillets of halibut or other mild white fish (use 1¼-1½ pounds of fish if using one piece)

½ cup Japanese bread crumbs (find in the Asian section of the grocery store)

½ cup chopped unsalted shelled pistachio nuts, crushed

1 tablespoon minced fresh garlic

1 tablespoon minced fresh herbs

such as thyme, basil, parsley or a combination

juice of one lemon

3 tablespoons extra virgin olive oil and more olive oil to coat fish

salt and pepper

*cut-up broccoli, cauliflower, or green beans

*If you want to make this a one-dish dinner,m add cut up vegetables in the baking dish around the fish and drizzle with olive oil, salt and pepper, and a sprinkling of your extra herbs.

Liberally coat fish with olive oil, salt and pepper. In a bowl mix bread crumbs, nuts, garlic, lemon, herbs, and 3 tablespoons of olive oil. Place fish in a baking dish and cover the top with the pistachio mixture. Bake in the oven at 450 degrees for 10 minutes (15 if the fish is more than 1½ inches thick). Serve with fresh herbs sprinkled on top and more lemon.

If you have extra of the nut and herb coating you can store it in the freezer in a zip-lock bag. Try it on chicken as well.

Olive oil is a great source of oleic acid, an omega-9 monounsaturated fatty acid, and mixed tocopherols (from vitamin E) which makes it good for the heart, the digestive system, and even good at fighting cancer.

Garlic is anti-inflammatory and is a great source of B_6. It is touted as an amazing medicinal plant providing protection from heart disease, some cancers, and infection.

CHAPTER 9

EMBRACE
NUTRITIOUS

**All things are permissible but
not all things are profitable.**

I seem to have raised a small posse of ingredient critics. My kids could convince someone it is a cardinal sin to eat anything with trans fats, hydrogenated fats, high fructose corn syrup, or artificial sweetener. I was once at a local store where they have gourmet coffee for customers to partake of in tiny cups. I rarely allow them caffeine (besides chocolate, *of course*), but occasionally I let them get a little taste of coffee with their cream and sugar. My littlest was reaching into a container for some sugar and picked up a pink packet of Sweet'N Low. The older one, who loves to be the boss, grabs her hand and says emphatically, "No, that's poison!" As my life goes, there was a properly coiffed and sophisticated lady pouring the contents of a pink packet into her coffee right beside us. I looked at her, shrugged my shoulders, and said with an ironic smile, "I don't know where they get these things."

A few times, when groceries were scarce or time was limited, I suggested the purchasing of one school cafeteria lunch. You would have thought I had asked them to kiss someone with cooties. Kids, like adults, have strong opinions when it comes to food.

∿∿∿∿

Let's examine how our own food opinions play out. Food opinions lead to food habits and food habits are the significant other in the weight-loss relationship (the calories in part). Have you noticed how incongruent our food habits can be? Often the same people with a tendency to overindulge, use artificial sweeteners and buy fat-free creamer. It's like the guy who always has a Diet Coke in one hand and a chocolate éclair in the other. We dwell so deeply in paradox, but our paradox has become predictable.

The crucial question here is, are our food habits working for us? Obviously not. This is where food philosophy comes in. In the last chapter, we looked at our views on food, and, hopefully, we are starting to reevaluate the way we view and, therefore, do food. So where are we missing it?

Socrates said, "Thou shouldst eat to live, not live to eat." As a self appointed food philosopher, I say, "Thou shouldst balance eating for health with eating for pleasure." Our weight issues reveal that we're not so much about eating for health and all about eating for either pleasure, convenience, or weight loss (and usually we flip-flop between the three). Eating for health, pleasure, and weight loss is wholly compatible if health is the main motive.

If convenience drives our food choices, weight loss and health usually go out the window and burgers and fries come in the drive-through window. Our habit of choosing junk food based on convenience, but its accessibility, omnipresence, and sometimes cost-efficiency do not change the fact that it is unhealthy and calorically costly. It's typically loaded with sugar, fats, or both, which may make it taste good, but those very ingredients also make it addictive and counterproductive to weight loss.

Besides eating for convenience, another unhealthy habit involves eating foods just because they promise weight loss. We've bought the line that if it is sugar-free, fat-free, and calorie free, it will set us free from our protruding misery. Guess what? It hasn't worked, it isn't working, and it *won't* work. Not only are these pseudo and chemically altered foods poor weapons in the battle of the bulge, they are fighting for the wrong team, contributing to the very problem they claim to fix. Our nutritional needs are not being met, and therefore, in an attempt to fulfill what our bodies really require (nutrients and energy) we are simply eating more of what it does not require. News flash: Our *bodies* were designed to eat *natural foods.* Our bodies know the difference in *nature's produce* and synthetic *products.* And we wonder why there is more and more disease.

Food can be healthy and delicious if we put the proper food philosophies into good food habits. So I am going to get on my food philosopher soapbox with some very simple and practical tools to change the way we think, shop, cook, and eat our food! The benefits are not confined to weight loss, but weight maintenance and improved health as well.

Soapbox #1: Ingredients Matter

Ingredients are either for you or against you.

It never ceases to baffle me that someone would choose a bag of potato chips with literally 22 ingredients (I don't make this stuff up) over a bag of chips with 2 or 3 ingredients: potatoes, oil, and possibly salt. What else do you need? What are those other 19 ingredients and how many of them are actually chemicals or "artificial food products"? So sometimes what's *not* in it, is just as important as what's in it. We need to face the fact: Ingredients are not neutral.

Food in its natural, unadulterated state is easier for our bodies to digest and more nutritious. But fresh food has been passed over for highly processed food filled with additives and preservatives. Since this generation is finally realizing that we are over-fat and undernourished, everyone is looking for a panacea supplement. It should be no surprise that supplements are not nearly as helpful as food because God put the right *mix* of nutrients in the fresh foods. Research is showing that in order for vitamin and mineral supplements to be fully beneficial they should be digested in concert with other absorption-enhancing nutrients...like those that occur in food naturally.

Even when it comes to fat we now know what some of us suspected long ago, that natural fats are better than processed ones. This is good news because I'm telling you to *occasionally* have some real butter, some really good cheese, and some ice cream *in moderation.* What is cheese, butter, or cream without fat? It's like saying "fat-free fat." It's a fraud.

We desperately need to get back to what I call "food integrity" and "food intuition." Food integrity involves evaluating what we are putting in our bodies, i.e., knowing the benefits and risks of the ingredients we are ingesting. When food is refined, processed, and artificial, it is at the very least lacking nutrition. A good way to gauge the integrity of a food would be to ask, "Did God make this food?" If the answer is yes, it passes the food integrity test. Another good question would be, "Is this food a nutrient-poor source of calories?" If the answer is yes, it doesn't pass the food integrity test. If we can take it one step further, "food intuition" means eating and paying attention to how certain foods make us feel in the short and long run! Our bodies, if we are attentive, literally crave much-needed nutrients. This is a long-term goal and benefit of eating well for years—it will come in time as your body adjusts to eating more natural fresh foods.

Remember: In general, the more natural state the food is in when consumed, the more naturally good it is for you.

Forgoing the Extras

In the *Super Size Me* documentary about a self-appointed guinea pig on a 30-day Mickey D's diet, Morgan Spurlock, the star and producer begins to feel terrible after a few days. Only a fix of french fries, Coke, sugar, and salt-filled food makes him feel better...temporarily. (Can you spell *addiction?)* Morgan's in a doom loop. The caffeine, salt, fat, and sugar are addictive in and of themselves. Researchers have studied the drug effects of these foods on the brain that perpetuate junk food addiction, and I cite some of the hormonal influences in the next chapter on portion control. Imagine the bang you get when you combine them. Fast-food companies are one step ahead of you, luring you into a cycle of addiction. You eat them, feel bad, and eat them again just to feel good, if only for an hour.

To get out of the addictive doom loop, we must ask ourselves some questions. What is our response to certain foods? Do we now feel hungry or satisfied, tired or energized, guilty or self-controlled? These things are highly pertinent to weight management. The amounts of extras added to our food, usually along the lines of additives, preservatives, food dyes, salt, sugar, high-fructose corn syrup, trans fats, hydrogenated fats, and a host of unnecessary, often harmful, and weight-loss sabotaging ingredients are mind-boggling when you stop and do the math.

As you know by now, I'm not a calorie counter, and I'm not suggesting that we dissect every calorie in a science laboratory, but we've thrown out all common sense when it comes to choosing our groceries and our dinner. We need to know what's in the food and equally important—what's not in the food. Instead of sugar-free (as in artificially sweetened), fat-free, calorie-free, and nutrient-free, we should be concerned with chemical-free, preservative-free, hormone-free, and antibiotic-free.

The Pink-and-Blue Challenge

Earlier I mentioned that ingredients are not neutral. They either help or hurt us and obviously the more natural, the better. Now I don't have a long food spectrum that I have created and specifically ranked everything in its place. But if I did I can tell you what would be at negative infinity. Artificial sweeteners. One simple challenge that I propose is to eliminate the little pink and blue packets. They are really best used to balance out a wobbly table leg (NutraSweet, Sweet'N Low).

Before I preach, let me confess that I used to drink up to a six-pack of Diet Coke a day. I wish I had known then what I know now. Some studies show that they can increase our appetite and cause insulin responses leading to weight gain, not to mention cancer and who knows what else. If I die after this book hits the press, please don't say, "See, she told us to eat healthy and look what all those health foods did for her." After the nonnutritive sweeteners and completely nutrient deficient foods I survived on, *I* will not be surprised.

Two of the primary ingredients in Equal and Sweet'N Low are

dextrose and maltodextrins, which can stimulate fat storage and elevate insulin. Aspartame contains methanol, a wood alcohol, which could potentially be metabolized into formaldehyde in the cells. I highly suggest weaning yourself off of them if you consume them daily and don't want a pickled brain.

Soapbox #2: Eat Nutrient-Dense Foods

This is the eat to live and eating for health side of the balance that is so gravely neglected, especially among those struggling to shed some poundage.

Years ago, when I was a grad student, an exercise physiologist told our class that food is just fuel for the engine or for activity, with carbohydrates being the preferred source for energy output. I was with him until he said a carb is a carb because they are all converted to glucose. Protein is protein because it will eventually be broken down to amino acids and used as a last resort for fuel. It really doesn't matter if it is oatmeal or a pancake. Not so fast, my mind shouted, and "What about nutrient density?" came out of my mouth, to which he replied, "Your brain doesn't distinguish nutrient density when it converts energy for use." I understood the point but was disappointed that he never revisited the differences in quality of food in regard to health, nutrition, and disease prevention. Your brain may not recognize the difference, but your body most certainly will over time.

All Calories Are Not Created Equal

Some foods are better for you than others based on their micronutrients (vitamins and mineral content, including antioxidants and phytonutrients) and their health promoting and disease fighting benefits. It is Common Sense 101. It doesn't take a biologist, physiologist, or a dietologist to understand that a baked potato is better than french fries. However, other examples might be surprising: Almonds have a denser vitamin content than pretzels and as mentioned above, nuts are being researched as aiding in the lowering of cholesterol and prevention of heart attacks. Wild salmon benefits our health more than many protein sources because of the beneficial omega-3 fatty acids (that's good "fatty" by the way). A serving boasts 1000 milligrams of EPA and 725 milligrams of DHA, the much needed omega-3s. Cold water fish has been shown to be beneficial in protecting against Alzheimer's, cancer, and heart disease. Even though olive oil has a little more fat than butter, (olive oil has 14 grams of fat per tablespoon and butter has 12 grams per tablespoon), olive oil is the superior choice. Butter has the saturated fat (solid at room temperature fat) which can raise LDL or "lousy" artery clogging cholesterol. Olive oil, with its monounsaturated fats, can actually help lower cholesterol (when it replaces the saturated fat in the diet). Easy does it, though (portion control—next chapter). Limit the amount to about one tablespoon a day to aid in weight loss. Avocados are another excellent source of monounsaturated fatty acids, as well as potassium, vitamin E, and fiber.

Some Fats Are Phat

Notice I intentionally mentioned some of the fattier foods to spur you to think about nutrient density as a part of healthy weight loss. If portions are kept in check, good fat—monounsaturated and polyunsaturated—can benefit weight loss. When it comes to fat consumption, moderation wins out over severe restriction as suggested by recent research. The metabolic processing of blood sugar, fatty acids, and cholesterol are dependent upon new fat from the food we consume. All of the hoopla aimed at getting us to reduce dietary fat during the last 20 years has promoted the consumption of nutritionally bankrupt, high-sugar, low-fiber foods, *un*coincidentally during the explosion of obesity rates. This is probably due to the idea that we crave sweet treats when fat is dramatically restricted. Fat provides satiety, which is crucial to weight control.[1] Good fats like those from olives, olive oil, cashews, almonds, avocados, fish, and soybeans benefit your brain and body. The bottom line about fat is to eat the natural ones in modest portions, combined with wholesome carbohydrates and quality protein.

I could cite a gazillion more studies but I'd rather tell you from personal experience that "Eating is believing." Those extra pounds I was carrying when I got married were probably partly because my body was healing from years of abuse and my metabolism had to slowly recover.

However, my very low-fat diet was not beneficial to my health or my weight. Eating fat-free and very low-fat carbs seemed smart. I was afraid of fat because of the abuse I had inflicted on my digestive system, so I basically avoided it like the plague.

Luckily, around this time I attended a Cooper Institute Fitness Specialist Certification program and had my cholesterol checked. To my consternation it was somewhat high considering I aspired to have immaculate (as in very low fat) eating habits. Interestingly enough I found myself lighter several years later with lower cholesterol without any intentional change in my eating habits. Weight training and possibly some minor changes in my Kardio might get an honorable mention, but I had done consistent Kardio for years.

After pondering the possibilities, I am convinced that adding nuts, seeds, avocados, and fish back into my diet made all the difference. I lightened up about fat and lightened up altogether. If we go too low in our fat intake it messes up the system. I'm a big proponent of balanced eating customized for our individual needs and lifestyles. It's all about eating the right things in the right quantities. And it's not that difficult to do!

Make Every Choice Count

So if all calories are not created equal, which calories should we choose? You can only take in a certain amount of expendable calories (energy) daily. When you are trying to lose weight, it makes even more sense to make your calories count in the nutrition department. That means getting the empty calories out. Sugar, high fructose corn syrup, and white flour are three prime examples of empty calories. Sugarholism is one of the major contributors to our nation's weight quagmire. In fact researchers are studying what seems to be a direct correlation between the increase in high-fructose corn syrup consumption and the increase in obesity rates in our nation. White flour is another nonnutritive, processed ingredient that could easily be replaced with wheat flour, which at least has some fiber. (A 50/50 mix of white and wheat flour for baking doesn't take away from the texture or taste.)

SOME USDA DIETARY GUIDELINES
FOR AMERICANS

Check this out to help get a grip on your sugar intake and limits: Look on chart 1 to find your age and daily calorie requirements, then look at chart 2 to find the maximum number of additional teaspoons of sugar you should have per day, then look at chart 3 to see the surprisingly high amount of sugar in some common foods.

For example, look at the average adult male. One Coke a day makes up half of the recommended added sugar consumption!

Chart 1
Estimated calorie requirements
(upper limit for an active person)

Chart 2
Guidelines for maximum daily added sugar consumption
(most of us are already getting plenty of natural sugar in the foods we consume)

Toddler (age 2 to 3)	1400	16 grams (4 teaspoons)
Teen boy (age 14 to 18)	3200	96 grams (24 teaspoons)
Teen girl (age 14 to 18)	2400	48 grams (12 teaspoons)
Adult male (age 31 to 50+)	3000	72 grams (18 teaspoons)
Adult female (age 31 to 50+)	2200	36 grams (9 teaspoons)

Chart 3
Sugar amounts in the foods we eat
(numbers vary slightly by brand)

Soda (12 ounces)	9 to 12 teaspoons
Sorbet, lemon (½ cup)	7 teaspoons
Sweetened yogurt (6 ounces)	7 teaspoons
Ice cream, chocolate-mint-cookie flavor (½ cup)	5 teaspoons
Barbecue sauce (2 tablespoons)	4 teaspoons
Tomato soup (1 cup)	4 teaspoons

Spend Your Allowance Wisely...

Your liquid calorie allowance, that is. Many beverages, pop in particular, have high calories and no nutrients to show for it. Besides, calories you drink do not tend to help satisfy appetite, just like eating an orange is better than drinking orange juice. The fiber and even the act of chewing make the orange more satisfying. Not to mention the heat pasteurization process it goes through to get to the shelf destroys some of the natural health benefits (enzymes).

Drinking water helps regulate body temperature and is vital to proper kidney function. Water is the superior weight-loss drink because it fills you up without adding calories. It also relieves fluid retention. Additionally, water increases metabolism, and especially if it is cold.

You read right, water revs the metabolic engine.

Researchers in Germany measured the resting metabolism of subjects before and after consuming water. Within 10 minutes of consuming about 16 ounces of H_2O, metabolism began to rise. After 40 minutes, the average calorie-burning rate of the volunteers was 30 percent higher and metabolism stayed elevated for more than 60 minutes. Over the long haul, water can make an impact on weight loss.[2]

Water, fizzy water, unsweetened tea, and tomato juice, because it is fairly low calorie, are some good beverage choices. I also add Emer'gen-C (small flavored packets of powder found in health food stores and some groceries) to water sometimes to give it flavor and boost vitamin C intake. (I like the raspberry.)

Super Foods Are Our Superfriends

If you don't know about the information explosion in the last few years regarding the amazing benefits of certain foods via the vitamins, minerals, and disease-fighting nutrients they possess, it's time to meet some Super Foods. These foods work overtime (behind the scenes) to help put you in control of your weight, your health, and your future.

There are so many foods being touted for their anti-cancer, anti-heart disease, cholesterol lowering, fat "inhibiting" properties that I would have to write a novel to discuss them all. Instead, I am going to list my top 15 picks with nutrition and health details. These are the *good unpronounceables*. You don't have to understand exactly how they work or memorize the vitamin contents, of course. Just know that they are working for your health and your metabolism and take it one step further: Eat them! I listed the Super Foods that boost weight loss as the top picks. Remember, I am not suggesting all or nothing or one size fits all but balance and incorporating some nutrient-dense foods into your daily life. Baby steps means changing a few things at a time. In the case of Super Foods, that means trying them and then incorporating the ones you like into your meals.

1. Yogurt or kefir: The potential health benefits of cultured dairy (related to the probiotic bacteria it contains) include improved intestinal health, lower blood cholesterol, and anti-cancer and immune-enhancing effects. Yogurt is a good source of protein, and, like other milk products, it is a great source of calcium. My favorite yogurt has 8 grams of protein and 30 percent of the daily recommended calcium per one cup serving. It is also a very good source of riboflavin and vitamin B_{12}, and a good source of other minerals such as zinc and potassium. An easy way to incorporate this into your meals is to throw some in a smoothie or you could also mix it with your morning cereal.

Weight-loss highlights: As you may have heard by now, calcium helps with weight loss. Studies show that calcium supplements are helpful, but they also show that it's even better to get calcium from dairy products. Overweight subjects who took a calcium supplement lost 26 percent more weight and 38 percent more body fat than the diet group who didn't. Another group got their calcium from dairy foods and lost an impressive 70 percent more weight and 64 percent more fat than the dieters who didn't get additional calcium. (Subjects consumed three to four servings of low-fat dairy, 1200 to 1300 milligrams of calcium daily.) Significantly, the fat loss from the tummy was substantial. Belly fat carries with it a greater risk for coronary artery disease than fat stored in the thighs and hips. Apple-shaped persons are at a greater risk than pear-shaped persons, which is why losing fat distributed around the waist is very good. Scientists are still studying the catalysts in calcium, but their suspicion is that calcium forces fat out of cells and into the bloodstream where it can be more rapidly utilized. No matter what the exact cause, an increase in dairy consumption is associated with a decrease in risk of being overweight.[3] Don't skimp on dairy, which is a diet temptation.

2. Green or black tea: Both are loaded with polyphenols, antioxidants that help prevent heart disease and cancer. They both contain fairly high amounts of vitamins C, D, and K and riboflavin, and good amounts of the minerals calcium, magnesium, iron, zinc, sodium, nickel, and fluoride. Green tea also may help prevent inflammatory diseases and stomach ulcers via the polyphenols, especially epigallocatechin gallate (and I didn't make that word up). More good news: Green tea may protect against Alzheimer's disease.

However, choose wisely when it's time for coffee or tea:

- *green tea:* 6 ounces has 8 to 16 milligrams of caffeine
- *black tea:* 6 ounces has 25 to 110 milligrams of caffeine
- *coffee:* 6 ounces has 60 to 180 milligrams of caffeine

Weight-loss highlights: Green tea may be useful as a glucose regulator, as in slowing the rise in blood sugar after a meal. We usually associate this with benefiting the diabetic, but when blood sugar is stable, it also helps minimize food cravings. A recent study published in the *American Journal of Clinical Nutrition,* indicated the ingestion of a tea rich in the catechins mentioned above, leads to both a lowering of body fat *and* of cholesterol levels, further validating the effectiveness of green tea.[4] I'll drink to that!

3. Flaxseed is rich in the omega-3 fatty acid, alpha-linolenic acid, as well as phytoestrogens, known as lignans. Omega-3 fatty acids have potent anti-inflammatory actions and help lower cholesterol. They also help reduce arterial plaque formation and may help reduce breast cancer. I put flaxseed on cereal, yogurt, and brown rice, but it is easy to add to almost anything and has a mild flavor. Flaxseeds are a good source of magnesium, potassium, manganese, and dietary fiber.

Weight-loss highlights: The research is out and fiber aids in weight loss by making us feel full on less calories. Adults should aim for at least 25 grams of fiber daily. In light of enhancing weight loss efforts I recommend 35 to 40 grams of fiber daily. Sprinkle flax on your favorite foods.

4. Broccoli or broccoli sprouts contain antioxidants that help prevent heart disease and glucosinolates that have anti-cancer effects. Broccoli boasts vitamins K, C, and A, plus folic acid and fiber. Broccoli sprouts, which are seedlings of the broccoli plant, are high in sulforaphane, another antioxidant that helps protect against cancer. Both broccoli and broccoli sprouts are low in calories and high in nutrients.

Weight-loss highlights: Fiber is your friend when it comes to weight loss! Mom was right—eat your broccoli.

5. Beans are a great source of complex carbohydrates, protein, and fiber. They are also a good source of folic acid and molybdenum. The major health benefit of beans is their cholesterol-lowering effect via fiber. Fiber in beans also prevents rapid rises in blood sugar. The antioxidants in beans, plus folic acid, vitamin B_6, and magnesium contribute to a healthy heart as well.

Weight-loss highlights: Fiber and fiber supplements can be useful in fighting fat. Fiber decreases insulin levels, enhances blood sugar control, and reduces the number of calories that the body absorbs. The most weight-loss-promoting sources are water-soluble fibers such as guar gum and glucomannan.[5] It doesn't benefit you to count beans if you don't eat them too!

6. Grapefruit: Low in calories, grapefruit is a good source of water-soluble fibers. It is also a good source of flavonoids, vitamin C, folic acid, and potassium. A whole grapefruit contains only 97 calories and 3.7 grams of fiber.

Weight-loss highlights: We've heard of the grapefruit diet, which involves consuming grapefruit ad nauseum, promising a ridiculous amount of weight loss in three months (over 50 pounds). The diet, which is mostly ludicrous, is on to something with the grapefruit. Grapefruit, it seems, *can* aid in weight loss. In one study of 100 obese participants, those who drank one cup of grapefruit juice or ate half of a grapefruit three times daily lost weight without adding exercise or intentionally cutting calories. The grapefruit groupies lost 3½ pounds in a 12-week period. Researchers suspect that grapefruit has obscure compounds that block enzymes involved in fat and carbohydrate storage. They may be baffled over the catalyst, but in the meantime, let's eat some grapefruit.[6]

7. Oats boast magnesium, iron, phosphorous, manganese, selenium, and calcium. They are also a good source of soluble fiber. Their ability to lower cholesterol, which has become a popular topic, is linked to the beta-glucan, a component of the dietary fiber. In persons with elevated cholesterol levels three grams of soluble oat fiber daily can lower cholesterol by 8 to 23 percent. That spells reduced risk of developing heart disease.[7]

Weight-loss highlights: We have already observed the potential weight loss associated with fiber (see above).

Tip—Buy plain rather than flavored oatmeal, which has lots of sugar. Instead, add a spoonful of peanut butter for flavor and protein combo. Stash individual oatmeal packs in your purse or desk drawer. In a bind for lunch? Just add hot water!

8. Soy (non-GMO, organic) is an excellent source of protein and molybdenum and a good source of iron, calcium, phosphorous, and fiber. Consuming soy can help lower blood cholesterol levels, and protect against heart attack and osteoporosis. (Some good sources: Of course soybeans, tofu, soy milk—or order the edamame next time you go for sushi.)

Weight-loss highlights: In one study, when dieters consumed 1200 calories per day in soy-based liquids vs. cow's milk, the soy-based products were more effective in aiding weight loss.[8] Incorporating soy liquids into your diet may help you fight fat, and it can add nutrition to your meals. So drink up!

9. Tomatoes are nutrient dense and low calorie, boasting vitamins C and K, and the now famous red carotene, lycopene. Lycopene has been extensively praised for its health-promoting ability, namely cancer protection. Breast, lung, colon, prostate, and skin cancer seem to be hindered by lycopene. It can also lower the risk of heart disease and cataracts. This is one exception where cooking actually enhances the nutrient value, so sauté away! Another great way to get a tomato a day is to make some salsa. And the onions in the salsa are a very good source of dietary fiber, vitamins C and B_6, and folic acid; the peppers have the ability to galvanize metabolism.

Weight-loss highlights: Some research has shown hot, spicy foods to benefit metabolism, though for a short period (we need all the help we can get). Peppers, of the spicy variety, mustard, and foods such as chili seem to shift your metabolism into a higher gear. In one study by British researchers, spicy food was shown to increase BMR (basal metabolic rate) by an average of 25 percent[9] (try the pico de gallo recipe, page 154). Turn up the heat and battle the bulge.

10. Walnuts are probably the most nutritious nut out there, although almonds deserve honorable mention. They are an excellent source of antioxidants, vitamin E, and the minerals manganese, copper, phosphorus, and magnesium. The press that walnuts are getting is based on their good, monounsaturated oils. Walnuts, an important food of the Mediterranean diet, are a great source of omega-3 fatty acids and alpha-linolenic acid (ALA). They have no cholesterol and contain protein and fiber. They have been studied for their cholesterol-lowering benefits and more specifically, they have been found to lower LDL (lousy) cholesterol. Though high in calories, they are an excellent "on the go" snack and can actually help stave off cravings. I eat some type of nuts or seeds daily. Almonds are also an excellent source of monounsaturated fats as well as protein, potassium, magnesium, iron, zinc, and calcium. (Did you know you could get calcium from almonds?) Grab a handful and off you go.

11. Quinoa (pronounced *KEEN-wah*): An excellent protein source, quinoa contains all the essential amino acids, making it an especially good protein source for vegans. It also boasts magnesium, manganese, vitamins B_2 and E, and minerals iron, zinc, copper, and phosphorous. It is also a good source of dietary fiber (fat fighter) and is known to be one of the least allergenic grains. I include it in my oatmeal, but it is a great rice, pasta, or bread substitute (see quinoa recipe on page 79). Give quinoa a try.

12. Salmon boasts protein and vitamin B_{12}, as well as potassium. Wild salmon (wild has more protein and less omega-6 fatty acids, which are the ones we seem to get plenty of, than farm raised salmon) is one of the fattier fish but before you go fataphobic on me, remember, we are trying to eat good fats and cut out the bad fats (trans, hydrogenated, and partially hydrogenated). Cold water fish helps protect against heart disease, Alzheimer's disease, and cancer. Salmon is an excellent source of the omega-3 fatty acids, EPA, and DHA. As you've probably heard, we get a lot more of the omega-6 fatty acids than the omega-3's.

Swim upstream and have some salmon!

13. Spinach is a great source of vitamins C and K, folic acid, and carotenes, including lutein. It is also a great vegan source of iron, containing double the amount as most other greens. Additionally, it is low in calories and boasts manganese, magnesium, and vitamin B_2. It promotes healthy eyesight and prevents cataracts because of the lutein, which is one of the many compounds in spinach that functions as antioxidants and anti-cancer agents. In studies involving stomach cancer, skin cancer, and breast cancer, intake of spinach has had a positive impact.[10]

Although I don't recommend spinach from a can, Popeye the sailor man was onto something (in addition to weight training) when he sang, "I'm strong to the finich cuz I eats me spinach." Spinach is powerful.

14. Blueberries are loaded with powerful antioxidants, including flavonoids, especially anthocyanidins. They also boast vitamin C, soluble fiber, manganese, vitamin E, and riboflavin. The anthocyanidins are responsible for their protection against Alzheimer's disease and their ability to improve vision. Blueberries also contain the same compounds in cranberries that help promote urinary tract health. By the way, researchers at Tufts University analyzed the antioxidant capacity of 60 fruits and veggies and blueberries got the top score.[11] Getting the blues is actually good for you.

15. Pomegranates: A single pomegranate delivers 40 percent of the daily recommended dose of vitamin C and may out-boast blueberries when it comes to antioxidants. According to a recent study, drinking pomegranate juice regularly can greatly reduce the size of atherosclerotic lesions, the fatty plaques that can block arteries, causing heart attacks or strokes.[12] The pomegranate and its beneficial properties which help fight heart disease and lower blood pressure have come from all the way around the world. In ancient Egypt, the rind was a remedy for intestinal worms and a juice was made from the pomegranate. Pomegranates are among the seven species listed in Deuteronomy, for which Israel is known. Even the chi-chi Hollywood types are into what is affectionately called

PJ, for pomegranate juice. Swap out your sugar saturated carbonated sodas for pomegranate and other natural juices and you're sure to see and feel a difference. I much prefer the seeds to the juice but give them both a try. Pomegranates are chock-full of good stuff.

Try to incorporate many of these supers into your meals for several months, and you will be amazed at the results. My tastes have changed dramatically in the last 15 years because I retrained my taste buds to appreciate wholesome foods, and my body is thankful. Paying attention to nutrient-dense foods has revolutionized the way I feel, the way I eat, and the way I maintain my weight.

MAKE IT *happen*

How to Build Your Food Integrity

I hope you will adopt some of the following food integrity principles, which are guidelines to help you make wise food choices.

1. Buy food in its most natural state.

2. Incorporate the nutritious Super Foods into your meals, especially the ones that promote weight loss.

3. Experiment with natural flavor enhancers such as lemon and lime juice, spices, and herbs, instead of salt, fat, and sugar. Even some culinary spices are getting rave reviews as health enhancers and disease fighters, such as turmeric, cinnamon, garlic, and ginger.

4. Start reading labels on all packaged foods (this part will probably be temporary).

5. Get the trans and hydrogenated fats out of your life!

6. Look for short ingredient lists on packaged foods (usually less is more).

7. Be suspicious of ingredients you can't pronounce, and cut out foods with chemical and artificial ingredients.

8. Stop adding sugar to coffee, tea, fruit, cereal, sauces, and everything imaginable and wean yourself off sugar-laden products and snacks.

9. Limit or cut out refined carbohydrates such as sugar, high-fructose corn syrup, and white flour, which have no nutritional value.

10. Drink (water, that is) to your health and weight loss.

MOM'S CHICKEN SOUP
Serves 4

2 boneless, skinless chicken breasts

6 cups chicken broth (low-sodium)

1 tablespoon olive oil (optional, with optional step)

3 tomatoes, chopped, with juice; or 8 oz. can of peeled, chopped tomatoes

1 cup diced onion

2 carrots, chopped

2 celery ribs, chopped

½ green bell pepper, seeded and chopped

2 tablespoons garlic

1 teaspoon turmeric

½ cup whole wheat macaroni (or other small pasta)

2 cups chopped fresh spinach

2 cups chopped fresh kale

½ cup fresh parsley, chopped

½ cup fresh oregano, chopped

salt and freshly ground pepper, to taste

Place chicken breasts in a large soup pot with the broth. Bring to a boil and reduce heat until broth is simmering. Simmer about 10 minutes, until chicken is cooked.

Remove the chicken and put on a plate to cool.

Optional step: In a separate saucepan, sauté tomatoes, onion, carrots, celery, bell pepper, garlic, and turmeric in the olive oil for about 2 minutes.

Skim the fat from the broth and return to a boil. Add the sautéed mix or add tomatoes through turmeric in the recipe to the soup. Simmer about 10 minutes until vegetables are soft. Add pasta and cook 6-8 minutes until al dente.

Chop chicken into small pieces. Add chicken, spinach, kale, parsley, and oregano to the soup and simmer another few minutes. Season with salt and pepper to taste.

Tomatoes have lycopene and vitamin C. Garlic has a good amount of B_6, manganese, selenium, and vitamin C and protects against heart disease and infection. Turmeric is an anti-inflammatory agent.

ROASTED VEGETABLES

vegetables

olive oil

salt

freshly ground pepper

Wash and slice a variety of fresh vegetables (see below for ideas). Preheat oven to 450°. Line a cookie sheet with foil and spray with cooking spray. Place the veggies on the cooking sheet and drizzle with olive oil. Season with salt and freshly ground pepper. Roast for 35-40 minutes until tender.

This is one of MiMi's (my sweet mother-in-law's) favorite ways to fix vegetables. It is fun to experiment with different vegetables each time you make it.

Choose from these great options:

tomato (Super Food)	bell pepper
sweet potato (loaded with carotenes)—unpeeled and sliced crosswise into ¼- ½ inch slices	onion
	Japanese eggplant—unpeeled and sliced crosswise into ½-inch slices
mushrooms	
okra	cabbage in 2-inch wedges
asparagus	broccoli (super food)
zucchini	brussels sprouts
yellow squash	

See above for the nutrition information on the Super Foods tomatoes and broccoli. Sweet potatoes are an excellent source of carotenes and a good source of vitamins C and B_6.

ALMOND-BUTTER SMOOTHIE
Serves 2

I make this when I don't have time to sit down and eat a meal because it is hearty and delicious. You can substitute peanut butter for the almond butter, too. For the sake of your blender, slice the ripe bananas and then freeze them in small zip-lock bags.

¾ cup organic reduced-fat chocolate milk

1 tablespoon almond butter

2 small frozen bananas (sliced)

½ cup plain low fat yogurt

½ teaspoon honey

Put all ingredients in blender and blend until smooth.

Almonds are high in calories and highly nutritious. They are a super source of protein, potassium, magnesium, calcium, iron, zinc, and vitamin E as well as monounsaturated and polyunsaturated fat. Almonds may help fight heart disease, cancer and, in moderation, the bulge.

Bananas are loaded with potassium and are soothing to the gastrointestinal tract.

Potassium-rich foods can help protect against heart disease and stroke.

CHAPTER 10
EMBRACE FRESH

You don't have to cook fancy or complicated masterpieces—just good food from *fresh* ingredients.

—*Julia Child*

Unless you're in food oblivion, you've probably heard these five words from every legitimate government health-promoting organization in the country: "Eat more fruits and vegetables." I would like to add one word to that: "Eat more *fresh* fruits and vegetables." One of the reasons I think we so often pass on the fruits and vegetables and opt for the French fries, chips, or cookies is because we are not eating fresh quality produce. Fresh food needs very little dolling up to make it palatable. Fresh broccoli, carrots, asparagus, and cauliflower are wonderful raw or lightly steamed with a little olive oil and sometimes a little salt or seasoning. Likewise, how hard do you have to work to make fresh watermelon, strawberries, blueberries, cantaloupe, or a Granny Smith apple taste good? God did His part. The key is getting it fresh and in season. Most people act like it is an impossible chore to eat fruits and vegetables. They get out an excuse list, which goes something like this:

1. "I don't like fruits and veggies."
2. "I don't have time."
3. "It's too expensive to eat healthy."
4. "I don't know how to prepare them."

Trust me—there are solutions to each of these common barriers, if you are willing to change.

Making Fresh Happen

Excuse #1: "I don't like them." You can retrain your taste buds. Start reincorporating some fruits and veggies into your daily meals. Experiment with variety. Get out of your comfort-food zone and try something new such as pomegranate, starfruit, leeks, or broccoli sprouts. You will find things you enjoy if you persist. To enhance the taste, try to shop for produce in season. For example, strawberries are at their peak spring through summer and tomatoes are generally better July through October. Cherry season is usually June through September. Oranges, though available year-round, are better in the colder months. Grapefruit is a good year-round fruit, and spinach is also good year-round (another reason to bring these Super Foods to your table). Another taste trick is to eat fruits and vegetables at room temperature to enhance the juiciness. This can be challenging if you live in a warm, humid climate like I do. I prefer room temperature produce, but I have learned that I must eat or refrigerate it on the day it's purchased. I try to take it out of the fridge one hour before I'm going to eat it.

Excuse #2: "I don't have time." The time issue is legit. Shopping more frequently is a part of eating fresh but remember the word commitment from chapter 1. If you are committed to changing the way you do food, in hopes of losing weight and improving your health, you will "make it (fresh) happen."

There are ways to save time, so let's brainstorm:

1. Buy veggies and fruits that don't even need to be cut up (for "on the go") such as baby carrots, apples, bananas, pears, blueberries (I eat them straight from the four-ounce carton). Even strawberries are easy to grab and eat.

2. Buy fruits and veggies already cut up (fast food gets a "fresh"-over).

3. Instead of buying the ingredients for a salad, visit the salad bar and pick one up. (I suggest going easy on the dressing or sticking with oil and vinegar.)

4. Prepare some "to go" baggies of fresh produce for the AM or PM when the munchies hit.

Also, keep in mind that frozen retains almost as many nutrients as fresh and is a useful alternative—but the taste is usually not the same.

Excuse #3: "It's too expensive to eat healthy." It is true that fresh, quality produce can be pricey, but all things considered, it's worth it. For example, the nutrition bennies can save you sick days, doctor's bills, diet bills, and even supplement bills (if you are eating some of the Super Foods such as oranges, you are reaping the beneficial micronutrients and can possibly forgo the vitamin C supplements). Think of it this way—maybe if you pay a little more, you will actually eat the broccoli that otherwise might sit in your fridge!

ANTIOXIDANT SCORECARD[1]

Food	Score	Food	Score
Blueberries, 1 cup	9019	Pecans, 1 ounce	5095
Cranberries, 1 cup	8983	Pinto beans, ½ cup	4983
Blackberries, 1 cup	7701	Sweet cherries , 1 cup	4873
Raspberries, 1 cup	6058	Black plum	4844
Strawberries, 1 cup	5938	Walnuts, 1 ounce	3846
Red delicious apple	5900	Green pear	3172
Red kidney beans, ½ cup	5569	Hazelnuts, 1 ounce	2739

Food	Score	Food	Score
Navel orange	2540	Pistachios, 1 ounce	2267
Red cabbage, ½ cup	2359	Green tea, 1 cup	2231
Russet potato, 6-ounce	2325		

In addition to "Eat more fresh fruits and vegetables," a six-word motto we would do well to repeat to ourselves daily, there are other important ways to make fresh happen. In order to eat fresh, you have to shop for fresh produce as well as dairy, meat, nuts, seeds, and fresh bread. If you want to find those fresh foods, stay on the perimeter aisles of the market. The processed foods are on the center aisles.

Excuse #4: "I don't know how to prepare it." After you shop fresh, you need to cook fresh. Following are some useful basics. (And of course you'll find straightforward recipes throughout this book.) When cooking vegetables keep in mind that the higher the temperature and the longer it cooks—the more you lower the nutrient value (heat kills the natural living enzymes). Here's the methods of cooking in the order that preserves more nutrients first: fresh, steamed, poached, blanched, boiled, baked, and fried.

The following cooking methods for making fresh happen save unnecessary calories and require very little effort:

1. Bake it ("put it in the oven for baby and me").

2. Steam it (suspend a perforated basket above simmering water on the stove burner).

3. Poach it (gently simmer in water or broth until tender).

4. Grill or broil it (placing food on the grill or broiler rack allows much of the fat to drip off).

5. Sauté it (in the skillet with broth, water, or a small amount of oil).

6. Roast it (see roasted vegetable recipe in the previous chapter, for example).

What's All the Organic Hype?

When I encourage people to eat more fresh fruits and vegetables, I will invariably get the question, "What about organic products—are they better?"

Organic products are experiencing exponential growth in the food business. Not long ago, organic availability was limited to the health-food stores and the farmer's market niche. Customers want options at mainstream grocery stores, and organics are even showing up at warehouse price clubs such as Costco. There are health and environmental benefits, but most people are choosing organics to reduce their exposure to chemicals in the foods they eat. Nearly two-thirds of U.S. consumers purchased some organic beverages and foods in 2005.[2]

Buying organic products reduces exposure to potentially harmful residues and other contaminants, and studies have confirmed that some organic veggies, fruits, and grains have higher antioxidant levels than their non-organic counterparts.[3] Organic simply means "living." "Organically Grown and Produced" indicates that it is grown without the use of synthetic fertilizers, sewage sludge, toxic pesticides, genetically modified organisms and made without artificial flavors and irradiation (see "Dirty Dozen" at end of chapter). As for meat and dairy, it's plastered across the organic labels, no growth hormones or antibiotics are used on the animals.

Even though one of my close friends said I should title this book *The Organic Girl's Guide to Weight Loss,* I'm not to the point of buying organically grown socks. When it comes to produce, beef, and dairy, though, organic potentially spells better for consumer health, and I want all the health I can get. My take—buy organic fruits and veggies when possible and wash non-organic produce well (I use Veggie Wash). As an avid organic shopper, I do sometimes suffer sticker shock when I purchase organic blueberries or strawberries. They can be twice the price of the standard ones.

How Can Organic Fit in the Budget?

First of all, you don't have to buy organic everything. *Consumer Reports* found that it pays to buy organic apples, spinach, peaches, beef, and milk to avoid chemicals in the conventionally produced versions, but seafood and shampoo had no organic advantages. (See the next page for some help on what to buy organic and what doesn't matter so much.)

Secondly, do some observing and find the most reasonable place to shop for organics. I've already mentioned that warehouse stores are now offering many organic choices. Even grocery store prices can vary dramatically. Hunt down a local farmer's market, if possible. I found a small one, less than ten vendors, that is on my beaten path once a week. Selection is limited but it's consistently cheaper than the natural foods grocery that I frequent.

Thirdly, buy a share in a community-supported organic farm and you will receive a weekly supply of produce and save substantially. (Go to www.sare.org and click on "for consumers" for a list of community-supported farms).

I hope this chapter inspires you once again to exchange the diet mentality that *is not working,* for the "food is good" mentality we have explored especially in these last three chapters. As you embark on a new way of moving and eating, applying some of these food integrity and fresh food principles, it will revolutionize the way you feel and positively impact your weight-loss attempts, helping you reach your goals.

MAKE IT *happen*

New Food Moves

1. Buy the freshest food you can find (which means shopping often and possibly finding a natural foods market, a farmer's market, or at least a grocery that has very fresh produce).

2. Eat organically as much as possible. Be aware of fruits and veggies with high pesticide residue.

3. Eat from a wide variety of colorful fresh fruits and veggies to get the nutrients you need.

"DIRTY DOZEN"

The following produce items tend to have a higher pesticide residue, based on data from the USDA. Consider buying organic from this list:

apples	peaches
bell peppers	pears
celery	potatoes
cherries	raspberries
grapes	spinach
nectarines	strawberries

"DOZEN'T" MATTER (AS MUCH)

The following items tend to contain little to no pesticide, meaning it is not as important to purchase organic:

asparagus	kiwi
avocados	mangos
bananas	onions
broccoli	papaya
cauliflower	pineapples
corn	peas

FRESH PICO DE GALLO

2 medium-size fresh tomatoes, stems removed and chopped

½ red onion, chopped

1 serrano chili pepper, stems, ribs, and seeds removed, diced

1 jalapeño chili pepper, stems, ribs, and seeds removed, diced

juice of ½ lemon or lime

¼ cup chopped cilantro

salt

freshly ground pepper

¼ teaspoon turmeric, dissolved in juice

Chop tomatoes. Prepare the chilis and dice finely. Be careful handling them and wash hands thoroughly with hot water and soap afterward. Set some seeds aside to add in later if you like it hot. Combine all ingredients, including salt and pepper to taste. Use as a topping for a mild fish or chicken or dip your blue corn chips (made with blue corn and expeller pressed oil).

Spicy foods rev the metabolic engine and turmeric is a powerful anti-inflammatory agent with anti-cancer properties and may protect against Alzheimer's (so don't forget to add turmeric).

GRAPEFRUIT-AVOCADO-ARUGULA SALAD

2 tablespoons fresh lemon juice

4 cups arugula

2 small avocados, pitted and sliced into about eight pieces per avocado

2 red grapefruit

1 pomegranate (optional)

½ teaspoon coarse salt

freshly ground pepper

2 tablespoons olive oil

lime wedges for serving (optional)

Place 1 cup arugula over each salad plate. Brush 2-3 teaspoons lemon juice over flesh of avocado slices.

Remove grapefruit sections with a paring knife. Work over a bowl to catch the juice. Put grapefruit segments in a small bowl and set aside. Reserve juice in bowl.

Add the lemon juice, salt, and tarragon to the grapefruit juice; season with pepper. Slowly whisk in oil. Add grapefruit sections and toss gently to coat.

Place avocado slices on the plates and top with grapefruit mixture and pomegranate seeds (if adding). Garnish with tarragon and serve with lemon or lime wedges.

Grapefruit is a good source of fiber, folic acid, vitamin C, and potassium. See the Super Foods information for pomegranates.

SPINACH STRAWBERRY SALAD

Serves 4

3-4 ounces spinach
1 cup strawberries sliced (or blueberries)
¾ cup thinly sliced mushrooms
¼ cup sliced almonds (toasted)

Dressing:

¼ cup extra-virgin olive oil
1 tablespoon balsamic vinegar
1 teaspoon honey
1 teaspoon organic ketchup (regular ketchup contains lots of high-fructose corn syrup)
1 tablespoon finely chopped onion (optional)

Mix salad ingredients. In a separate bowl, mix dressing ingredients, reserving the onion. This makes extra dressing so pour the dressing you need into a separate bowl and mix in the onion. Drizzle some dressing over each salad. (Extra dressing will keep in fridge for about a week.)

My girls love this salad (I leave the onion out of theirs).

Spinach and almonds have the omega-3 fatty acids. Spinach has B, C, and E vitamins, calcium, iron, magnesium, and zinc. Strawberries and mushrooms add more antioxidants and phytonutrients.

GREEK SALAD

Serves 6-8 as an appetizer or side salad

Dressing:

½ cup quality extra-virgin olive oil

¼ cup fresh lemon juice

1 teaspoon Dijon mustard

2 teaspoons finely chopped fresh oregano

1 teaspoon chopped oil-packed anchovies

In a medium bowl, whisk together all ingredients. Let sit for 15 minutes to allow flavors to merge.

Salad:

3 cups arugula, washed and dried

3 medium firm-ripe tomatoes, cored and chopped

2 firm ripe avocados, sliced

1 cucumber, chopped

½ red onion, chopped or sliced

1 cup kalamata black olives, pitted and quartered

8 ounces firm feta, chopped

coarse salt

freshly ground pepper

Place the arugula on a large platter and arrange the other ingredients in sections on top of the arugula (do not mix ingredients). Whisk the dressing and drizzle over the salad or serve in a pitcher with the salad.

The tomato is packed with beta carotene, lycopene, and vitamin C. Avocados are a terrific source of monounsaturated fats, and they are packed with potassium and fiber.

FRUIT SALAD DRESSING

Covers 6-8 bowls of fruit

3 medium oranges

1 small to medium avocado, mashed

1 large banana or 1½ small bananas, mashed

2 tablespoons Greek-style or lowfat yogurt

½ teaspoon cinnamon

1 tablespoon organic flaxseed oil

½ cup ground almonds (optional)

Combine the freshly squeezed juice of the oranges with the avocado, banana, yogurt, and cinnamon in a food processor and process until smooth. Grind the almonds (could use a coffee grinder).

Drizzle 3-4 tablespoons of the sauce over each bowl of fruit and sprinkle about 2 teaspoons of the ground almonds on each serving.

I have used this over blueberries and pineapple chunks or sliced apples and bananas. It is mild enough to be delicious over whatever fruit is in season.

Oranges have a high vitamin C content and good amounts of B vitamins. They contain strong antiinflammatory properties. Avocados, though high in fat, contain the good unsaturated fatty acids and plenty of potassium. Flaxseed oil has a myriad of health benefits because of its abundance of omega-3 essential fatty acids.

EASY DINNER SALAD
Serves 4

4 cups mixed greens

1 cup radicchio (optional)

2 tablespoons olive oil

1½ teaspoons balsamic vinegar

freshly ground black pepper

1 cup toasted walnut halves

Wash the greens and radicchio and pat dry with a paper towel. Place both in a bowl. In a small bowl, whisk together the olive oil and vinegar, and pour over the salad. Add a bit of black pepper if desired. Add the walnuts and serve.

Walnuts are incredibly nutrient-dense, boasting both omega-3 fatty acids and alpha-linolenic acid (ALA). They contain protein, fiber, and plenty of antioxidants and minerals.

Radicchio and other members of the endive family boast only about one calorie per leaf and eight calories per cup because of the high water content. They are a good source of fiber and vitamins A and C.

CHAPTER 11

EMBRACE SATISFACTION

You won't give me something
that gives me more pleasure than You.
Because You've created nothing
that gives me more pleasure than You.

—from "You Created" by Caedmon's Call

The story is told that a reporter once asked billionaire John D. Rockefeller how much it would take to satisfy a man. His provocative response was, "Just a little bit more." We live in one of the most materially saturated countries in the world, and yet our mantra is still *more, more, more*—more money, more power, more stuff, more square footage, more freedom, more options, more time, more techno-toys, more pleasure, and more *tres leches*. We feel entitled to muchness, and overabundance is our common lot. And there seems to be a general, unspoken consensus that more of everything that is "good" is better.

More Is Less

Last fall I taught a self-esteem series to a group of young women. The theory behind the whole self-esteem movement is simple: If you received a lot of praise from your parents growing up, you'll have high self-esteem; and if you didn't receive a lot of praise from your parents growing up, you'll have low self-esteem. In other words, the more people shower praise on you, the healthier and more secure you'll be. It *seems* true enough, right?

In my research for the series, I came across some enlightening information from clinical psychologist John Rosemond. He referenced a study that exposed the fallacy that children need a lot of praise to build self-esteem. In this study, five-year-olds were taken in two groups of ten to an activity area. Art supplies were provided there, and the children were told to create something as several teachers oversaw them. The first group received a lot of praise for their art project, while the second group did not. The next day, all of the children who were abundantly praised avoided the art table like it was quicksand, and the second group spent most of their time there. Rosemond's conclusion was that too much praise can have a negative effect when it is evaluative in nature. Evaluative praise is the expression of favorable judgment about another person, and the focus is often on performance: "Johnny, you did a superb job on your artwork!" The child might internalize perfectionistic standards that he eventually feels he can't meet, leading to feelings of inadequacy. He also notes: "Like sugar, praise can be habit-forming. Children who are praised either excessively or evaluatively often develop a dependence on outside approval."[1] Who would've ever guessed that too much praise can have negative consequences?

Take a look at technology. I doubt anyone would argue its benefits to society; however, it is driving some of us crazy these days, not to mention the fact that it's getting way over our heads. I have some technocratic friends that have such a complex lighting system for their house that they can barely make it work. Instead of simply flipping the light switch on, it takes about three swift moves and the touch of a safe-cracking artist to illuminate things while they eat dinner. I'd say this is technology gone awry.

How about caffeine? I, someone who visits the java dealers daily, must acknowledge that too much coffee is bad. Some caffeine studies point to the benefits (trust me, I have them memorized), citing the antioxidants, the positive effects on attention and mood, the quickening of reaction time, the possible short-term memory enhancement, and last but not least, its classification as an ergogenic aid—meaning it can boost athletic performance. Studies involving cycling and running reveal that caffeine can actually prolong the time to exhaustion. However, caffeine has a stimulant effect that can cause gastric distress, irritability, nervousness, and insomnia. It is a diuretic too, which means it can be dehydrating. I must admit I can tell a huge difference in my workouts when I am caffeinated versus overcaffeinated.

And in case you hadn't heard, too many vitamins and minerals can actually have negative effects on our health. For example, iron is vital for oxygen and the blood, but too much iron is toxic and can cause distress to the liver or kidneys. Our bodies must have zinc too, but interestingly enough, we need very little of it for ideal functioning. Too much fiber can cause stomach problems, too much soy could be carcinogenic, too much wine leads to drunkenness, and the list goes on.

Overwhelmed with Choices

And what about too many choices? I am flabbergasted by the 40,000 products lining the average supermarket's shelves these days. Just consider all those shelves lined with sugar, fat, and fake ingredients wrapped in colorful packages. Seriously, do we really need 10 choices of pretzels and 15 oatmeal options? The cereal section is particularly daunting. A whole aisle is devoted to boxes with kid-luring photos and large print, advertising all of the vitamins and health benefits of a particular cereal. If you look a little closer and see the sugar content, most of them are glorified breakfast candy. True, they have added vitamins back in, as evidenced by the words *fortified* and *enriched,* but why did they have to take them out in the first place?

I personally get overwhelmed by the infinitude of choices, which is why I tend to shop at stores that have an emphasis on the peripheral aisles. Outer aisles are typically stocked with fresh fruits, vegetables and herbs, fish, low fat dairy products, and often nuts and seeds. And guess what? If you shop these aisles, you don't have to read as many labels to figure out if it will benefit or *unfit* your body. And if you want to eat lean and healthfully, the good news is that the choices are already limited for you. For example, there are possibly 100 different yogurts to choose from in the dairy section at your typical grocery store. The healthiest yogurt, because it is not filled with added sugar, is plain, low-fat yogurt (you can add fresh fruit yourself). At healthy markets, there are only a handful of these to choose from. (Go back to chapters 9 and 10 if you need to review tips for healthy shopping.) The main point here is that too many choices in the grocery store often add up to too many calories and unhealthy additives in our bodies.

Portion Distortion Wins the Title

Speaking of too many calories, clearly our input is exceeding our output, and this is mainly because our portions are *disproportionate* to our needs. In the competition for what's making Americans so fat, portion distortion wins the heavyweight title. But what, or who, is really to blame for what appears to be this sudden obesity epidemic?

Many dub the fast food industry as the culprit. In the eye-opening documentary *Super Size Me,* Morgan Spurlock eats from McDonald's menu for 30 days straight, which obviously sets him on a fast track to obesity. I think (and yes, I watched the whole thing) his point was to lead us to the conclusion that obesity is a direct result of the rapid growth in fast food availability and consumption. I would be comfortable if the emphasis was on consumption, but I'm afraid the blame was more on availability. Do you see the difference? I would agree that availability does present a huge problem, but it goes much deeper than that. We'll address this issue in a moment.

For now, we can all agree that the fast food business is booming, and the portions are growing along with it. Not only are the meals on the menu usually high in fat, calories, salt, and sugar, but they are also larger in size than in years past. For example, a large order of McFries weighs about six ounces now, as compared to the two and a half ounces in 1960. The former small Coke is now the "kiddie" coke, and the large Coke now boasts 32 ounces, with over 20 teaspoons of sugar!

Morgan does his fair share of portraying the greedy side of this mega-million dollar industry, and it's hard to argue against him. Don't let the miniscule price increase it takes to *supersize* fool you. Fast food joints are making more money on their mega-sized servings, meanwhile edging out the competition, and keeping the McFans coming back. It's all about cost-efficiency. Welcome to corporate America, where the dollar dominates, and, unfortunately, this is at the price of health and quality—at least in terms of food.

CONSUMPTION QUOTES

Let's not be naïve to the moneymaking intentions of even our favorite food and beverage companies. Eric Schlosser's book *Fast Food Nation* dishes out some pretty alarming information. For example, he cites a Coca-Cola deal negotiated for Colorado Springs School District 11. The contract specified an annual sales quota: "School District 11 was obligated to sell at least seventy thousand cases of Coca-Cola products a year, within the first three years of the contract, or it would face reduced payments by Coke."[2]

But instead, only 21,000 cases of Coke products were sold between the elementary, middle, and high schools. Beverage sales were falling short, and the principals of the schools were warned that school revenues could be affected. The result: Coke machines would be placed in more visible spots on the campuses.

Pointing (Chicken) Fingers

Was Morgan right after all in saying that these big corporations are the chief blame-bearers? If so, then what do we do? Picket? Tell ourselves that because it's a big, faceless "they," suing for an exorbitant amount of money is okay, even *right*? Many have taken that route, with lawsuits aimed at McDonald's, Coca-Cola, Pepsi, Kelloggs, and the like, for "making" everyone fat, from Junior to the neighbor's cat. In fact, so many "fat" suits have been filed or threatened against these corporations that the government has finally decided to step in: "The U.S. House of Representatives overwhelmingly approved a bill Wednesday to ban lawsuits by obese customers who say they became overweight by eating at fast-food restaurants," reports the CNN Washington Bureau.[3]

Let's revisit Morgan's documentary for a moment, and we'll find something very interesting in regard to our weight-problem blame games. One of his rules in the supersize me experiment was: "I have to super-size it if they ask me." I "*have* to," he said. Rather revealing, isn't it? The implication is that we don't have a choice. Like moronic sheep we can do nothing but fall in line in the following fashion. They say: "Would you like the *super-d-duper* meal deal for 35 ½ cents more?" We say: "BAAA! Why not?" It's like the mega-deal stores, where we can't pass up an opportunity to buy 100 Styrofoam cups even though we only need 20. Why not, right?

The answer to the *why not* is because the excess just goes to waste or takes up space. And when this happens, we are desperate to make "them," whoever "they" are, the whipping boys. After all, why should *we* have to say, "No, thank you," or bother to take our hard-earned money elsewhere, in some cases?

Passing the Buck

The truth is, our shirking of responsibility has grown to epic proportions. This is dangerous for all of us, but it is especially dangerous for our children. Not only are American adults getting fatter, but "rates of overweight and obesity among children in the US have doubled and even tripled in some areas over the past 25 years. Depending on definitions, anywhere from one in seven to one in four children and adolescents are overweight."[4] When I look around at the children in pre-kindergarten through fifth grade who already have a weight problem, my heart hurts for them. Are we setting them up for a predisposition toward obesity, a diminished quality of life, and a host of associated diseases? Who is this "we"? No one wants to take the blame. I remember seeing a T-shirt one time that said, "Chocolate makes your clothes shrink." Humorously telling.

I have to be honest, when it comes to the growing problem of a nation of overweight children, I look no further than the parents. Most parents would gladly blame Ronald McDonald, sweets, fast food, marketing schemes, daycare workers, teachers, birthday parties, school cafeteria food, grandparents or the nanny (this is a favorite), and even the child, in an attempt to pass the buck.

Another popular scapegoat is genetics. But long-term studies of overweight children show that the degree of excess weight at puberty, along with the degree of excess weight in the family, and *not* your genes, are the two most significant predictors of body weight in adulthood. Please allow me to clarify: "Environmental factors"—family lifestyle, not genetics, are the major culprits in overweight children who graduate to obese adults.[5] Role modeling an active lifestyle to our children is important, and so is what we are feeding them. These factors pave the way for a healthy future or an unhealthy one, for good habits or bad ones, for an appropriate weight or an inappropriate one. The good thing is, it's never too late to start making healthy choices for our children, but we must first accept the responsibility.

A friend from out of town called me about her five-year-old son who is already noticeably overweight, asking for some advice. I have to admit, though I could hide it over the phone, I was incredulous when she commented: "He just really likes food." I am all astonishment! Most often, a child's weight problem begins as a parental problem.

Before we can even think about setting limits for our children, however, we need to set them for ourselves. No one else can do it for us. Make no mistake about it—basic economics tell us that companies are not going to discourage over-consumption. The meal-deal pushers, the aunt whose self-esteem hinges upon your eating more of her chocolate cream pie, and the co-worker who wants a partner in his croissant bingeing, are not going to change or disappear. And fast-food restaurants aren't going anywhere either. The omnipresence of temptation when it comes to over-indulgence demands that we put into practice saying: "No, thank you," "No more," and just, "No!"

No One Dares to Utter the "G-Word"

Gluttony is not a very popular word. In fact, we'd rather call someone a beached whale than a glutton. It's sounds so deprecating and judgmental, much more so than the words obese, fat, and overweight, which we throw around like categories on a job application. Why is it that I have never heard anyone say: "She's a glutton"? Because we don't like to draw cause/effect conclusions when the causes are in our control.

Webster's defines gluttony simply as the habit or act of eating too much. It could also be defined as consuming more than we require. Scripturally, gluttony is associated with laziness and idolatry,[6] but instead of associating our weight problems with these *sinful* things, we cite things like fast-food consumption or video games. Or we feel we must conform to our politically correct climate and allow that "metabolically and genetically, some people are predestined to be overweight." I agree that in *some* cases weight problems can be associated with predispositions toward obesity, but in general, our weight problem is about our eating problem, coupled with our sitting problem.

WHEN YOU SPLURGE, SPLURGE!

Food should be good, and food should be pleasurable, and there should be times of feasting and celebration with food. But, in reality, we have made times of feasting and celebration null and void because we are feasting constantly. There is no longer a distinction between "partying" and eating. We see business meetings, family meals, dinners at home, and dinners out with friends, as the time to indulge, without realizing that these are everyday occurrences. Thanksgiving, Christmas, and special anniversaries are no different from any other meal. Why should we look forward to them or be thankful? Ho-hum, it's just another feast. Although we appreciate the vacation days, we don't anticipate the food as much as generations before because we get a glut of it all the time. Abundance has lost its richness.

Remember the short-term dieting mentality we discussed in chapter 2? We'd be wise to transfer that short-term idea to our feasting. In other words, the times of indulgence should be the exceptions, and the practice of self-control should be the rule. Let splurging truly live up to its name. It's much more enjoyable that way!

What Really Satisfies

One problem when it comes to food and the comfort and pleasure we associate with it, is that we can no longer distinguish between physical hunger and emotional hunger or satisfaction and gluttony. As you will recall from the previous chapter, "fake" food is not meeting our nutritional needs, so we are simply filling our bodies with more of it, in an attempt to be satisfied. In other words, we are eating, but we are not feeding our bodies. Sometimes our overeating is not so much about gluttony as it is about malnutrition. This is the nutrition-deficit side of wanting more. And you may be surprised to know that this is a problem for overweight people just as it is for the hungry.

There is also the emotional and spiritual side of wanting more food in an attempt to gain feelings of security. The phrase "soul food" takes on a whole new meaning now, doesn't it? The truth is, many of us have put food at the center of our souls and have placed our delight in satisfying our sweet tooth, fat tooth, or salt tooth. And the more we eat, the more our bodies begin to require in order for the "feelings" of satiation to come. The other sinister agent in the area of overindulgence, however, is that the more we get, the more we want. Portion control is out of control because we seldom practice self-control. We feel a sense of entitlement to indulge every desire to the fullest, but many of us wouldn't know true fullness if it punched us in the gut. So how do we know what true fullness is? There are two primary ways.

Just Filling the Void

First, we need to recognize that many of us have gluttonous hearts that won't be satisfied even by overeating. Often a hunger for love is at the core of our need for "more." Another root cause of our gluttony is not trusting God as provider, so we search for security elsewhere. We feel we must "store up" pleasures on earth because they will not always be there. The size increases mentioned above are not simply a reflection of corporate greed; they also are the results of a gluttonous society. We are not very good at practicing frugality in the face of food.

There is a void in our soul, and we look to the people and things around us to fill it. Too much food is one of the most prevalent excesses of our time. It is an unending pursuit, often reflecting our lack of contentment in God, who alone can silence the cry for more. From the depth of our spiritual lack, we look to food for abundance and satisfaction. But God is saying this to us:

> Ho! Every one who thirsts, come to the waters;
> And you who have no money come, buy and eat
> Come, buy wine and milk
> Without money and without cost.
> Why do you spend money for what is not bread,
> And your wages for what does not satisfy?
> Listen carefully to Me, and eat what is good,
> And delight yourself in abundance.[7]

The abundance here is not in food but in God. The abundance of God is true sustenance. Consider the elements that represent God's sufficiency and (bodily) presence. The symbols of this meal, the bread and wine are simply the fruit of the earth and the fruit of the vine. They are bare and basic, and they call us to a deep acknowledgement that the abundance of God is enough to satisfy our deepest longings.

We need desperately to start being satisfied with the abundance of God instead of looking elsewhere. King David wrote, "The LORD is my shepherd; I shall not be in want."[8] "I shall not be in want" here means literally, "I lack nothing," and was birthed out of the recognition that God is everything we need, and the presence of God satisfies our deepest hungers. Apart from God, we will just be singing with Mick, "I can't get no satisfaction," no matter how much we consume.

Chemical Rewards

In addition to our emotional and spiritual reasons for overeating, there are actual chemical reasons for this tendency. Foods like fries, potato chips, cookies, and ice cream—which are the main overeating "agents"—disrupt the body's appetite-regulating system, causing you to want more and thereby thwarting your weight-loss attempts. Most people don't binge on carrots and celery. When you eat, "fullness" hormones are secreted, including leptin and insulin, which signal us to cease ingestion. This finely tuned system is disrupted by foods packed with sugar and fat, which creates a false hunger cue. Additionally, the taste experience is far more intense than that of healthful foods, leading to the secretion of dopamine, serotonin, and possibly other feel-good chemicals. Instead of being hungry, we are craving a chemical "high" or reward.[9]

I think this is exactly what happened to Edmund in *The Lion, the Witch, and the Wardrobe,* when the White Witch introduces him to Turkish delight. "At first Edmund tried to remember that it is rude to speak with one's mouth full, but soon he forgot about this and thought only of trying to shovel down as much Turkish delight as he could, and the more he ate, the more he wanted to eat…" What the queen knew and Edmund didn't, was that "anyone who had once tasted it would want more and more of it, and would even go on eating it till they killed themselves."[10]

Sugary, fried, and caffeine-laced foods, much like Turkish delight, are nonnutritive and addictive and should be eaten only occasionally and in small amounts for this very reason.

Less Is More

What exactly is our responsibility? Ultimately we are responsible for what and how much we eat. When it comes to portion control, we have to take a cue from "less is more." My 80-year-old Bible study teacher has a great sense of humor. I heard him point out that less is more when it comes to wives and consequently mother-in-laws. Of King Solomon, who had a plethora of wives, not to mention concubines, he asks, "Can you imagine having to keep all those women happy?" Poor Solomon could have learned from the less is more philosophy.

We too could learn from the concept of "less is more" and save ourselves untold calories, while benefiting our eating habits across the board. Take margarine and its popularity. If I gave a taste test to 20 people, I doubt that anyone would choose margarine over butter. So why do we use it? To save calories and fat? Maybe, but I would wager that we choose margarine for the same reason we choose many diet, low-calorie, low-fat, and low-carb foods…so we can have *more.*

However, we are fatter as a country even though we are consuming less fat now than in previous years. We've traded fat for refined carbohydrates, and we are consuming fat-free products like they are calorically comparable to water. We're still overeating, though. Let's keep it real. A pat of butter or a drizzle of olive oil, both natural foods (though that word has suffered abuse lately), can enhance a piece of bread, or some asparagus, or popcorn, like drowning them in margarine could never do. A dollop of whipped cream (don't worry—I'm going to define dollop) on hot chocolate can be a tasty addition, whereas a cup of low-fat Cool Whip overwhelms the cocoa flavor and overwhelms our stomach. A handful of raw nuts is often more satisfying than 20 pieces of celery. Bread pudding is incredibly rich and, therefore, delicious in moderation, yet it is nauseating in excess. What's it going to take to turn the tide of an overweight nation?

Let's Get Down to Portions

What we need is to get highly practical about weight control by implementing self-control and learning portion control. There are no totally off-limits foods, but limited portions of all foods, especially the more fat-laden and sugary ones. You can eat any food you want on occasion, as long as you are vigilant about the amount. You can have a meal that is a feast when this is the exception. All things in moderation. When I go to someone's home for dinner, I don't inquire, "Is this meal preservative-free, trans-fat–free, food-coloring–free, hormone-free, antibiotic-free, certified organically grown, and nutrient-dense?" Typically, I eat what is set before me. However, I have control over how much I eat because I have a little piece of fruit in my pocket called self-control. "But the fruit of the Spirit is love, joy…and self-control."[11]

How can we reduce our consumption, also called downsizing, as opposed to supersizing? I've already bashed calorie counting for numerous reasons. A more pragmatic approach is to relearn servings so that we can control our portions. Americans have fallen prey to portion distortion, and we are underestimating how much we're eating and overestimating the recommended serving sizes for many foods. Have you ever wondered how many average cookies you could eat to match the calories in that deluxe-size bakery cookie? If you haven't, you need to. When you choose the biggest bagel from the bread tray, you are thinking one bagel equals one bread serving, when in actuality, it could count for three or four servings from the bread group. You just blew half your bread allowance for the day. People tend to eat in units, which can easily translate to overconsumption, based on the size of the unit. You've got to stop eating for two, unless you're expecting.

Just look at the labels on some common commodities like Coke. The nutrition facts tell you the calories and sugar content of 8 ounces of Coke, even though you're holding the 20-ounce bottle, thinking it is one serving. Who buys an 8-ounce can or bottle of Coke? Or an even more appropriate question is, who buys a 20-ounce Coke and drinks 8 ounces? When I really want to convince someone to kick the soda habit, I bring a 20-ounce Coke bottle with nothing but the sugar in the bottle. A 20-ounce Coke has about 18 teaspoons of sugar in it, shedding new light on the term "coke addict."

It seems we have lost our sense of "intuitive eating" and rely too heavily on visual input in relation to portions. In other words, the amount of food we consume during a meal is highly influenced by vision. One study involving eating behavior of subjects while blindfolded versus not blindfolded revealed a 22 percent decrease in food intake when blindfolded: "Despite a smaller amount of food consumed when blindfolded, the reported feeling of fullness was identical to that reported after the larger meal consumed without blindfold."[12] My hope is that eventually we can relearn fullness, but first we must train our eyes to evaluate portions. The American Institute for Cancer Research website has some useful information about the New American Plate. Their model encourages us to aim for meals made up of at least two-thirds vegetables, fruits, whole grains, or beans; and one-third or less animal protein. But how big should the plate be?

The popular food guidelines tool is the pyramid. I like both the Mayo Clinic Food pyramid and the American food pyramid because these recommend a daily number of servings from each food group and they define serving sizes, which is critical to our supersized guestimations. For example, on the Mayo Plan, a serving of milk is 1 cup and a serving of rice is ⅓ cup. Become familiar with 1 cup, ½ cup, and ⅓ cup units and teaspoon measurements for fat control. In getting to know servings, measure your food when you dine at home for about a week, or until you feel confident about eyeballing amounts. At this point you can graduate to the common objects method of measurement that follows the serving sizes in the sidebar below:[13]

WHAT IS A SERVING?
WHAT DOES A SERVING LOOK LIKE?

Food	Serving size	Looks like (visual cues)
Chopped vegetables	½ cup	½ of a baseball
Raw leafy vegetables (for example, lettuce)	1 cup	one baseball
Fresh fruit	1 medium piece	one baseball
Fresh fruit	½ cup chopped	½ of a baseball
Dried fruit	¼ cup	one golf ball
Pasta, rice, cooked cereal	½ cup	½ of a baseball
Ready-to-eat cereal	1 ounce, which varies from ½ cup to 1¼ cup (check label)	varies
Meat, poultry, seafood	3 ounces (boneless cooked weight from 4 ounces raw)	deck of cards
Dried beans	½ cup cooked	½ of a baseball
Nuts	⅓ cup	level handful
Cheese	1 ½ ounces (2 ounces if processed)	four dice

Sizes of a few vague portion terms:
- What is a *dollop*? A lump, blob, or generous standard spoonful of a semiliquid substance.
- What is a *pat* (as in butter)? A small, flat, square individual portion (a little smaller than a sugar packet).
- What does *"use sparingly"* mean? It means use a very small amount—just enough to enhance the taste or texture.

Practical Tips for Diminishing Portion Sizes

Following are some general, across-the-board hints.

Don't be famished when it's mealtime. This is always what triggers out-of-control eating for me (when I have forgotten to eat lunch and, therefore, I am famished by the time dinner rolls around). Instead, have a handful of nuts, some carrots and celery with hummus (see recipe), a few slices of apple with a spoonful of peanut butter, a piece of cheese, yogurt, a cup of chips with black bean salsa (see recipe), or any quality snack, preferably with a mix of the macronutrients (protein, fat, and carbohydrates) to stave off hunger, even if you are within a couple of hours of dinner. Let me tell you a huge secret that might be helpful. Appetite is not a perfect science. Sometimes I am voraciously hungry and I end up overeating before dinner or when I am cooking dinner. Instead of beating myself up about it (I'm into grace, remember?), I will have a snack supper. I want to sit down with my family and enjoy their company and be a part, but I am no longer in need of a three-course meal.

Remember, no one and no situation forces you to overeat. Adjust your intake by opting for one or two side orders and feel no regret. Apply this to any meal. At the end of the school year last May I had two luncheons to go to back to back. Instead of drooling over the food at the second luncheon, I simply ordered a small salad and fizzy water, ate slowly, and thoroughly enjoyed the fellowship. I have a friend who blames the pastries and croissants at corporate meetings for her overeating. I wholeheartedly agree that most companies do not provide healthy options when it comes to meetings. Pack a mix of almonds, dried fruit (I like cranberries because they have a high antioxidant count), and walnuts (omega-3s) or pecans in a snack bag and bring it to work on meeting days (¼ to ½ cup should tide you over).

You can feel full on smaller portions by eating more water- and fiber-rich foods. Fruits, vegetables, soups, and salads qualify as lower-density foods that satiate. In a trial involving women, Barbara Rolls, professor of nutrition at Penn State University, "found that lowering the calorie density of their daily diets by 30 percent and reducing their portion sizes by a quarter caused them to eat 800 fewer calories in a day and still feel satisfied."[14] By simply reducing portion size and calorie density, we can lose weight without going hungry while eating nutrient-dense food.

Dish it out, and choose snacks wisely. One of my clients reduced the portions her family eats in the home by serving dinner on her salad plates. If you sometimes eat from the bag or the box, or even worse the carton (as in ice cream), start dishing it into small bowls. Don't eat meals in front of the TV. If you frequently snack in front of the television, start drinking water or herbal tea or allowing yourself some healthful fruits and veggies. When the munchies hit while I'm in front of the tube, I like to bring a bowl of blueberries, a thinly sliced apple, a bowl of raw veggies, a handful of mixed nuts (high in calories but cholesterol lowering and stave off hunger in small amounts), or a small bowl of organic unbuttered popcorn. It's not as tempting to binge on these foods. My kids love to eat edamame (soybeans from the shells) while they watch a show.

Practical Portion Control When Dining Out

First of all, view eating out as an experience and a chance to relax, instead of an interruption from the more important aspects of the day. Most of the people I talk with eat out a lot, which as we have seen can be portion trouble. Here's how to do it without sabotaging your weight-loss efforts: It's difficult to eat well at fast food, burger, and pizza joints, and Mexican food can be challenging because of the chips alone. Patronize restaurants with healthy options, even for take-out. Avoid buffet style restaurants and places that adhere to the bigger-is-a-better-value trend. Try to retrain your mind to think about quality over quantity. Americans spend significantly less on food compared to the French. We want it cheap and we're paying a big (bigger) price in compromising our health and fattening up our waistlines.

Also, you don't have to compete for the clean-plate award. If you are concerned about waste (this from a girl who recycles everything), consider how "waistful" it is to overeat—you will wear it on your waist. Besides, you can get more bang for your buck with some savvy strategies. When you order, order a half portion or a lunch portion if it is offered. Split an entrée with your dining partner or doggie-bag half of it up front and save the other half for another meal. Another trick of the lean is to order a salad or soup up front in order to prevent overeating or have them both as a meal (watch the dressing, as dressings are up to 100 percent fat and some have a small amount of carbs). In short:

- Split an entrée with your dining partner.
- Order a half portion and save calories and *dinero*.
- Doggie bag half of it up front.
- Choose restaurants that emphasize quality over quantity.
- Avoid buffets—too little quality, too much quantity.
- Order a soup or salad up front.
- Order dressing on the side.

Plan ahead and leave room for dessert instead of eating until you feel sick. (On rare occasions, our family will have a milkshake for an early dinner and a substantial and healthy snack later, instead of eating dinner and then topping it off with something incredibly rich, fattening, and filling.)

Portion Control at Home

- Don't skip breakfast. Eat a substantial one. You are breaking your 10-to-12 hour fast and waking up your metabolism.
- Don't skip lunch. Eat a solid one.
- Don't skip dinner. Eat a reasonable one.
- Snack between meals if you get hungry, and keep it healthy. Smaller, more frequent food consumption is actually good for your metabolism.
- Try to avoid eating in front of the TV. (Rather, savor your food by eating slowly.) I can count on one hand the number of times in over 15 years of marriage I have had dinner in front of the TV.
- Don't put food on the table. Serve plates and sit down.

It takes about 20 minutes for the stomach to respond to "full."

- Keep high-fat and high-sugar foods out of sight and healthy snacks within reach (I keep cereal, fruit, and nuts out on the counter).

- Mix carbs, protein, and fat as often as possible to avoid sugar lows and cravings (this is easier than worrying about the glycemic count of a carrot or a banana).

YUMMY HUMMUS

- 1 15-16-ounce can garbanzo beans, drained (liquid reserved) and rinsed
- ¼ cup roasted, chopped red bell peppers
- 3 tablespoons lemon juice
- 2 tablespoons cilantro (optional)
- ¼ cup tahini
- 3 tablespoons olive oil
- 1 teaspoon Bragg Liquid Aminos (alternative to soy sauce)
- 3 cloves garlic
- ⅛ teaspoon turmeric
- ⅛ teaspoon black pepper
- ⅛ teaspoon cayenne pepper
- 1 tiny red Anaheim pepper, chopped with seeds (optional for spicy hummus)

Process the beans, peppers, and lemon juice in food processor. Add the rest of the ingredients, cover and process until smooth. Add some bean liquid if necessary. Refrigerate and serve with veggies (I like to serve it with celery sticks, carrot sticks, slices of red bell pepper, or blue corn chips).

Garbanzo beans (chickpeas) are a great source of molybdenum and a good source of fiber, folic acid, and manganese. Garlic and turmeric are anti-inflammatory agents.

GUACAMOLE

Serves 6

- 2 small avocados (or one large)
- 1½ teaspoons lemon juice
- 2-3 tablespoons finely chopped onion
- ⅛ teaspoon salt
- ¼ teaspoon chili powder
- ¼ teaspoon cumin powder
- 1 small chopped tomato
- freshly ground pepper to taste

Mash avocados in a medium bowl and stir in the remaining ingredients. Serve with crudités or blue corn chips.

Avocados are an excellent source of monounsaturated fatty acids, as well as potassium.

Tomatoes have lycopene, a tremendous antioxidant.

CHUNKY BLACK BEAN SALSA

1½ cups black beans, cooked and drained (can also use canned)

1 cob of corn, cooked, kernels sliced off the cob

1 red bell pepper, seeded and chopped

2 tablespoons fresh cilantro, minced

1 tablespoon fresh parsley, minced (optional)

1 jalapeño pepper, seeded and chopped

1 tablespoon fresh lemon juice

1 tablespoon fresh lime juice

salt and freshly ground pepper

1 firm avocado

Combine all ingredients, reserving avocado. Add salt and pepper to taste. Cover and chill about an hour (or up to 24 hours). Before serving, chop avocado and add to the mix. Serve with large blue corn chips. (The chip needs to be substantial to hold the salsa.)

Beans are a super source of cholesterol-lowering, blood sugar stabilizing fiber and antioxidants.

STARBURST FRENCH FRIES

2 red bell peppers

2 yellow bell peppers

2 orange bell peppers

(can use 6 red bell peppers if preferred)

Core and slice bell peppers. Sprinkle with seasoning (see below). Left-over seasoning will keep in the pantry for up to a year. Cook at 450° for about 35 minutes or broil until blackened. The peppers will turn out crisp and candied.

This is a great substitute for french fries, a delicious snack, or a colorful side dish. This recipe was given to me by my friend Toni.

Seasoning:

2 teaspoons salt

⅛ teaspoon freshly ground black pepper

¼ teaspoon cayenne pepper

⅛ teaspoon chili powder

⅛ teaspoon garlic granules or powder

Bell peppers are low-calorie and incredibly nutrient-dense, boasting vitamin C, beta-carotene, vitamins C, K, B_6, thiamine, and folic acid. They have extraordinary antioxidant levels. Red bell peppers also contain lycopene.

MARY ROSE CHICKEN

I used to call this Rosemary Chicken, but my youngest, who has a way with words, would request Mary Rose Chicken for dinner.

4 boneless, skinless chicken breasts	½ cup freshly squeezed orange juice
4 teaspoons freshly chopped rosemary	¾ cup dry white wine (or wine substitute)
½ teaspoon salt	¼ cup maple syrup
½ teaspoon freshly ground black pepper	3 tablespoons olive oil

Mix rosemary, salt, and pepper in a small bowl and rub on both sides of the chicken breasts. Set aside.

Bring wine and orange juice to a boil in a small saucepan. Reduce heat slightly to a low boil for 5 minutes and stir occasionally. Stir in maple syrup and boil for 5-6 more minutes, stirring frequently until the mixture thickens slightly. Set aside.

Heat olive oil in a large skillet over medium heat. Add chicken breasts and cover. Sauté for 5 minutes (until browned on each side). Pour syrup over chicken (may bubble). Reduce to simmer, cover, and cook for about 10 minutes.

I serve this with my easy brown rice (see recipe below).

Orange juice as we all know is a super source of vitamin C, and it is also a super source of flavanoids. Additionally, it is a good source of B vitamins (1, 2, 6, folic acid, and pantothenic acid) and carotenes. Olive oil is a fab source of omega-9 oleic acid and contains mixed tocopherols (a good source of vitamin E).

MY EASY BROWN RICE

Yield: approximately six cups

2 cups uncooked brown rice (I use long grain)

2 ¼ cups (filtered) water

2 cups green tea

½-1 teaspoon salt

2 teaspoons extra virgin olive oil

1 teaspoon Bragg Liquid Aminos (alternative to soy sauce)

Combine rice, water, tea, and salt in a medium to large saucepan. Bring to a boil. Add olive oil and liquid aminos and stir a few times. Cover with a tight fitting lid. Reduce heat and simmer for 40 minutes. Remove from heat. Let stand for 5-10 minutes.

If you want a sweet-tasting rice, omit the liquid aminos and add 2-3 teaspoons of maple syrup.

I cook with green tea in place of water or soup stock all the time. I love the mild flavor, and I like to think my kids are getting something extra in their rice (they won't drink green tea).

Green tea is full of vitamins C, D, and K as well as good amounts of calcium, magnesium, iron, and zinc.

CHAPTER 12

THE NEW WAY TO KISS

The only joy in the world is to begin.

—*Cesare Pavese, novelist*

I must confess that my husband has married a lot of women. I don't hold it against him, though, because when I say "married" I am talking about conducting the wedding ceremony. You see, Ben is the associate minister at a rather large church and has performed umpteen weddings in the last 20 years. We have more than three weddings and a funeral every weekend, not to mention that I have worn the beloved bridesmaid's dress in 13 weddings. There is one part of the wedding ceremony that I particularly like. No, it's not the cake, it's the kiss. Don't we all anticipate the kiss? How will they kiss? How long will they kiss? Will they miss? We love the kiss.

∾∾∾∾

Practically speaking, it's time to KISS. It's time to implement the KISSing part of our new body philosophy, which requires a shift in priorities. When I was writing this book I said no to almost everything optional for a few months. It was therapeutic for my guilt-driven conscience. When I wasn't writing or thinking about writing, I was spending time with my family. I prayed, cooked, went to church, did laundry, and wrote. Nonessentials were eliminated from my schedule. My kitchen was usually a mess, my car was usually a mess, and I would have been a mess if I hadn't followed through with some important habits that I have developed over the years, namely exercising, eating well, and sleeping well.

Every season of life is about ordering priorities. Staying faithful to what we deem as important is being true to God and true to ourselves. Try as we may, we can't do it all and usually there are serious consequences for our attempts (failed marriages, out-of-control kids, and an out-of-shape body are some of the most glaring examples of trying to do too much and saying yes too often). The pursuit of doing it all is as elusive as 36-24-36. Listen, friends—we've got to set boundaries that protect our priorities and make exercise and eating well happen. Let the weight loss begin.

Let the Weight Loss Begin with SAM

We need to do a few things before we are ready for the KISSing part. First, get with a friend or significant other and discuss any lifestyle barriers that might hinder your weight-loss success and problem solve. Two heads are better than one, and articulating the things that need to occur in order for you to reach your goals both gets them on the table and provides some accountability, which we will explore in more detail in a minute. Next, set some goals. At the risk of sounding acrostic obsessed, which I will be in this chapter, remember the acrostic SAM. Your goals should be Simple, Attainable, and Measurable.

Simple: As you already know in any KISS plan, simplicity is vital. This plan involves four simple things that can change your weight forever.

Attainable: Set realistic goals. I suggest setting some goals that will assist *both* health and weight loss, as opposed to making weight loss your only goal. For example: "I am going to start eating oatmeal for breakfast, and I am going to walk four days a week." Write down those goals and record your progress in the journal at the end of the chapter. It will be encouraging to see that you have taken steps toward making these things a permanent part of your life.

Then, establish your realistic weight-loss goals. Write down your current weight, a short-term weight-loss goal like four pounds this month, and a long-term goal keeping the one to two pounds weekly rule of thumb in mind. An energy intake reduction of 500 calories per day, the calories in a typical five-ounce muffin, coupled with an increased energy output of 500 calories per day equals about two pounds of weight per week, the maximal recommendation by those of us who believe in lasting weight loss. One or two pounds a week is realistic, and it is slow enough that the weight loss is most likely from fat and not merely water.

Measurable: Weigh yourself about twice weekly while trying to lose. Check your progress with your goals in your eating and exercise journal (see an example of an exercise journal in the Resources section).

Learning the New Way to KISS

KISS, the old acrostic for "Keep It Simple, Sweetheart," applies to the simplicity of exercise and eating well. We have enough complex issues to ponder: nature versus nurture, why bad things happen to good people, predestination versus free will, the Trinity, and so on...Those things are mind-boggling complexities. Exercise is not complex, and it works for everyone—old, young, male, female, Jew, and Gentile.

The other meaning of KISS is my simple lifestyle acrostic for weight loss and weight maintenance. It's easy to remember and practical to live by:

- K*ardio:* cardiovascular exercise
- I*ntake:* ingest fresh food
- S*trength:* strength training
- S*pirit:* Spiritually grounded weight loss—asking for God's help, strength, guidance, and blessing in making lasting changes

"K" Stands for Kardio

Back to KISSing and the first letter K. The K, as you've noticed (I promise I know how to spell cardiovascular) stands for Kardio. I've emphasized the why and this is the how.

This Kardio prescription, based on ACSM guidelines, Kenneth Cooper's recommendations, and years of my own application, is broken down for you in another easy to remember acrostic FIT: FIT stands for Frequency, Intensity, and Time, three crucial aspects of your exercise and weight-loss goals. Intensity and time or duration of exercise determines the total energy expenditure during your training session. I am recommending a training intensity of 60 to 85 percent of your maximum heart rate (HRmax—see next page). The lower your initial fitness level, the lower the initial level of intensity should be. For example, if you have not been doing any exercise, even an intensity level of 40-50 percent of HRmax could be helpful.

Other factors to be considered include preferences for exercise and personal goals. ACSM recommends 20 to 60 minutes per Kardio session, a doable goal that will be highly effective when it comes to weight loss. Again, initial fitness must be considered and goals set accordingly. It is possible that 20 minutes of continuous exercise needs to be progressed toward. In the hopes of preventing undue fatigue and injury my Kardio program outlined below progresses modestly and consistently giving the body time to adapt. Frequency, intensity, and time are interrelated variables and can be manipulated according to your fitness level, preferences, and lifestyle. However, within these recommendations are minimums to be worked toward and maintained for life in order to lose weight, keep the metabolic fire stoked, and maintain the desired weight.

Memorize these guidelines and incorporate them into the seams of your life, and you will be amazed at the changes in your body and your attitude toward weight loss.

Here are the Kardio recommendations:

- *Frequency:* 3 to 6 days weekly
- *Intensity:* in your target heart rate range (60 to 85 percent HRmax); or using perceived exertion, between 4 and 15 Borg Scale (see page 186).
- *Time:* 20 to 60 minutes

The FIT recommendations above, combined with smart intake, which we discussed in chapters 9 through 11 (quality control and portion control), weight training, and prayer and meditation are the method I propose for achieving and maintaining your weight-loss goals forever.

Figuring Out Your Target Heart Rate

First you need to figure out your THR range. *THR* stands for *Target Heart Rate,* and it is a way of monitoring intensity. In order to reap the health, fitness, and weight-loss benefits of cardiovascular training, you need to be exercising at a certain intensity. (This is where Kardio and lifestyle activity usually part ways!) The easiest way to determine your THR is to find your carotid (neck) or your radial (wrist) artery, count the beats for 10 seconds during exercise, and multiply by six to determine your one-minute effort. (Or count the beats for 30 seconds and multiply by two.) In other words, stop exercising briefly and place the tips of the index and middle fingers over the artery and press lightly. Avoid using the thumb. Start counting on a beat, with "zero." This will determine your exercise heart rate and can then be compared to your goal range.

Some machines have heart-rate monitors (pulse detectors) built in. Or you can bite the bullet and purchase a heart-rate monitor. (I used one when I was pregnant.)

Here's the formula for estimating maximum heart rate (HRmax):

$$HRmax = 220 - Age$$

And the formula for estimating target (training) heart rate:

HRmax x exercise intensity (60 percent, 70 percent, and so on)

For example, a 30-year-old's maximum heart rate would be
  HRmax = 220-30 = 190
And the THR would be
  190 x 60 percent = 114 (lower end of THR)
  190 x 70 percent = 133
  190 x 85 percent = 162
In other words, THR range for a 30-year-old would be between 114 beats per minute and 162 beats per minute.

Here is a helpful chart:

Age	Target Heart Rate (THR): Zone 60% to 85%	Predicted Maximum Heart Rate
20	120-170	200
25	117-166	195
30	114-162	190
35	111-157	185
40	108-153	180
45	105-149	175
50	102-145	170
55	99-140	165
60	96-136	160
65	93-132	155
70	90-128	150

As you can see, this chart provides a range from 60 percent (the lower end of your training heart rate) to 85 percent (the high end). If you are just starting, or starting over, when it comes to Kardio, stick to the lower end of the THR range.

Another common method of assessing intensity is the Borg Scale, which is based on perceived exertion or self-assessment. (Though this is a common method, I don't recommend it for those who have never exercised consistently. Obviously, perceptions are not as accurate as formulas.)

The Borg RPE Scale (for intuitive exercisers)

6	No exertion	14	
7	Extremely light	15	Hard (heavy)
8		16	
9	Very light	17	Very hard
10		18	
11	Light	19	Extremely hard
12		20	
13	Somewhat hard		

Using this scale, a good goal would be to feel like you are working out somewhere between 11 and 15 for cardiovascular conditioning corresponding to your target heart rate range.

With due respect to Mr. Borg, a more user-friendly measurement of perceived exertion that we use in the exercise industry is a 1-to-10 scale—from no exertion to extremely difficult. Take your pick, but remember, intensity matters.

What Activities Qualify As Kardio Anyway?

Here are some activities that qualify as Kardio, aerobic, or steady-state exercise. Aerobic exercise (Kardio) is different from anaerobic exercise (such as weight training) in that it is continuous and rhythmic (both use large muscle groups). These activities could accommodate all fitness and skill levels simply based on intensity adjustments. The list below is not exhaustive, but this gives you some ideas to choose from.

Any endurance-oriented exercise that uses the large muscle groups in a rhythmic continuous fashion is considered cardiovascular or aerobic exercise and can be effective and efficient in initiating caloric expenditure. If you have joint pain, swimming or walking are good choices.

- walking
- hiking
- swimming
- cross-country skiing
- jogging
- running
- biking or cycling
- aerobics (called cardiovascular conditioning when including cardiovascular orientation)
- spinning (group-oriented stationary cycling)
- Stairmaster (machine)
- dancing
- stair-climbing (free-form or machine-based)
- rowing
- rope-skipping

When applying the FIT principle to Kardio, remember that a slow and modest increase in weekly exercise (or every other week, as shown below) should be attainable and allow the body to progress and the mind to adapt.

It would be unwise and uncomfortable to go from no exercise to exercising most days a week. These recommendations are reasonable goals to progress toward. I start beginners off with 15 minutes of aerobic exercise three days a week. However, if you cannot complete 10 to 15 minutes of continuous exercise, start with 5 to 10 and build on that. It is equally important, especially for adherence, that you exercise at an appropriate level, meaning a level that puts you in your target heart rate range and that you can sustain for the duration of the session.

After incorporating these workouts successfully into every other day or every third day for two weeks, make an assessment. How does my body feel? Am I ready to progress? If you feel good about progressing, see intermediate level or add two minutes to every other week for the next few weeks. As you can see, there is no rush to progress to the desired minimums because I propose that you do this for the rest of your life! Before you start, there are a couple of things that will help you ease into exercise.

Getting Started—The Warm-Up

Even though the verdict is out on stretching and the best time to stretch is after you warm your muscles up, I still find that people want to stretch right off the bat when it comes to exercise. Because your muscles are not warmed up you could potentially overstretch, as in injury. You will want to start any form of exercise with a 5-to-10-minute warm-up. A warm-up is exactly what it sounds like in that it should elevate your core body temperature. It also prepares the body by increasing the blood flow to the muscles and joints. The warm-up basically gets the engines revved for whatever you are about to do, which is why I suggest doing that very activity at a lower level for 5 to 10 minutes before you crank up the effort (put the pedal to the metal). If you are going to power walk, warm up with 5 minutes of semi-brisk walking, preparing your heart and the walking muscles. If you are about to lift weights, do some type of Kardio for the warm-up, such as power walking, jogging, cycling, Stairmaster, EFX, treadmill, or any rhythmic exercise at a fairly easy level. Warming up before you pick up the dumbbells or pick up the pace prepares the muscles for stretching. Take about 5 minutes to stretch including four or five stretches for major muscles. Ease into each stretch and hold for 30 to 60 seconds and move on or repeat if tightness is evident. Here are several ideas to get you stretching:

Stretches

Calf stretch (the large muscles on the back side of the lower legs): Face a wall with your feet a little further than arms length away from the wall. Place your hands on the wall and with your heels on the ground, lean forward with your hips until you feel the stretch in the calf muscles. You will get a better stretch in each calf if you focus on one leg at a time.

Quadriceps stretch (the large muscle of the upper thigh): Stand sideways to a wall, with one hand on the wall for balance. With the other hand reach for the ankle or the foot (on the same side of the body as your hand) and pull the heel up toward the derriére. Switch sides and repeat.

Hamstrings stretch (the large muscles on the back side of the upper legs): Stand upright with arms hanging to sides and bend forward, reaching toward the toes. Feel this stretch up the back of the legs.

Butterfly stretch (for the inner thighs): Sit on the floor with your back straight and your knees out to the side. Join the feet so that the soles are touching. Place your elbows just above the knee joint and gently press downward stretching the inner thigh and muscles around the groin.

THE KARDIO WORKOUT

BEGINNER level—If you are starting over, if you are new to exercise, or if you have not been exercising a few days a week for a consecutive 10 minutes. Example:

Week 1   Frequency: Monday, Wednesday, Friday (or day one, two, three)
Intensity: lower end of THR range (60 percent)
Time: 15 minutes

Week 2   F: Monday, Wednesday, Friday
I: lower end of THR range
T: 15 minutes

Week 3   F: Monday, Wednesday, Friday
            I: lower end of THR range
            T: 16 minutes

Week 4   same

Week 5   F: Monday, Wednesday, Friday
            I: lower end of THR range
            T: 17 minutes

Week 6   same

Week 7   F: Monday, Wednesday, Friday
            I: lower end of THR range
            T: 18 minutes

Week 8   same

Week 9   F: Monday, Wednesday, Friday
            I: lower end of THR range
            T: 19 minutes

Week 10   same

Week 11   F: Monday, Wednesday, Friday
            I: lower end of THR range
            T: 20 minutes

Week 12   same

Congrats! You made it to 20 minutes of continuous exercise. This is considered a great base amount of time for Kardio. Look back through your exercise journal (in Resource section), and see how you have set goals and achieved them. Look at your progress, and pat yourself on the back. You are on your way to becoming a lifer! Then assess your new weight and re-evaluate your goals.

INTERMEDIATE level—You have been exercising two or more days a week fairly consistently for eight weeks or more—for 10 to 20 minutes per session—and you are ready for a bigger challenge and a bigger payoff. Example:

Week 1   F: Monday, Wednesday, Friday
            I: middle of THR range (60-70 percent)
            T: 20 minutes

Week 2   same

Week 3   F: Monday, Wednesday, Friday
I: middle of THR range (60-70 percent)
T: 22 minutes

Week 4   same

Week 5   F: Monday, Wednesday, Friday
I: same
T: 24 minutes

Week 6   same

Week 7   F: Monday, Wednesday, Friday
I: same
T: 26 minutes

Week 8   same

Week 9   F: Monday, Wednesday, Friday
I: same
T: 28 minutes

Week 10 same

Week 11 F: Monday, Wednesday, Friday
I: same
T: 30 minutes

Week 12 same

Wow! You made it to 30 minutes of continuous exercise three days a week. Look back at your exercise journal and pat yourself on the back if you stuck to this most weeks. You are setting goals and achieving them.

ADVANCED level—You have been consistently exercising two or more days a week for 8 weeks or more—for 20 minutes or more per session—and you are ready for a bigger challenge and a bigger payoff. Example:

Week 1   F: Monday, Wednesday, Friday, Saturday
I: middle to high end of THR range (70-80 percent)
T: 30 minutes

Week 2   same

Week 3 F: Monday, Wednesday, Friday, Saturday
I: middle to high end of THR range
T: 33 minutes

Week 4 same

Week 5 F: Monday, Wednesday, Friday, Saturday
I: same
T: 36 minutes

Week 6 same

Week 7 F: Monday, Wednesday, Friday, Saturday
I: same
T: 39 minutes

Week 8 same

Week 9 F: Monday, Wednesday, Friday, Saturday
I: same
T: 42 minutes

Week 10 same

Week 11 F: Monday, Wednesday, Friday, Saturday
I: same
T: 45 minutes

Week 12 same

Congrats—You made it to 45 minutes of continuous exercise! If you still need to lose weight or want to enjoy even more fitness benefits, add another day of exercise, increase the intensity to an intermediate level, or continue to increase the time of each Kardio session at a reasonable progression up to 60 minutes. This is where it gets fun and individualized by you.

In acknowledging that we are all unique, flexibility, freedom, and personality preference should be built in by you. Manipulate the variables in accordance with your personality and lifestyle (type A's might choose shorter, more intense bouts of exercise) always keeping in mind the minimums. I rarely put in an hour workout, mainly because of schedule, preference, and personality. My hard-core running friends call me a minimalist. I jokingly tell them I already have a religion. I do just what it takes to stay in running shape. I put in one day of pretty intense training every week almost year-round and add another speed workout if I am training for something specific, but most days I just enjoy easy running and even power walking (which is a nice opportunity to pray while getting some exercise).

Figure out what you like about working out and build on that. If you love to change it up, try Stairmaster one day, power walk outside another, or take a Kardio class one day to reach your frequency goal. If you need accountability, hire a trainer to assist you or recruit a friend to join in the pursuit of weight loss, fitness, and even fun. Some music lovers can't exercise without their iPod tunes. Regardless of what helps you get your groove on, find ways to make Kardio fun and you will make it happen. Several weeks into your new exercise program I hope the minimums of three days, 20 minutes in your THR zone are unforgettably imprinted in your microchip. Think: 20/3/in the zone.

Kardio is first in the acrostic because a little bit of Kardio goes a long way. To put it another way, if you blow it in the eating department and miss a weight-training workout…Kardio has a magical way of compensating.

"I" Stands for Intake

Since I've already stood on my food soapboxes, I'm just going to recap some of the crucial aspects of intake:

- Remember to balance eating for weight loss and health with eating for pleasure.

- When it comes to food, think fresh, as in "eat more *fresh* fruits and vegetables."

- Food integrity includes paying attention to the ingredients in the foods you are consuming.

- Nutrient density matters because you can only consume a certain amount of food. Make those foods work for you by choosing plenty of Super Foods. List the Super Foods you consume daily in your food journal in the Resource section.

- Last but not least, take control of portions—and you will be well on your *weigh*.

~~~~~

When KISSing, remember that the "K" stands for Kardio, the "I" stands for Intake, and the first "S" stands for Strength training. So let's get lean *and* strong!

"S" Stands for Strength Training

It is a good idea to start your strength- or resistance-training regime specifically with weight training before you go off doing your own "plank" (a rather challenging Pilates pose). Get familiar with your muscles and which ones you are utilizing for certain exercises. The muscle groups that should be worked in a balanced weight-training program include *quadriceps, hamstrings, gluteals, abductors, adductors, chest, back, shoulders, biceps, triceps, and core.* Working these 11 groups, as discussed in chapter 6, will help build muscle and prevent muscle loss, thereby benefiting metabolic rate and aiding in weight-loss effort. All the benefits we looked at are yours for the lifting.

Since muscular endurance, rather than muscular strength, should be emphasized with a weight-loss program, lighter weights and higher repetitions are better than heavy weights with relatively few repetitions. This will be better understood after we examine sets and repetitions.

Sets and Reps

Sets and reps are a way of counting how many times you perform a given exercise. For example, one set of ten reps is one set of the same exercise performed consecutively ten times. Sets and reps are divided to allow you to work the muscle, give it a short rest, and work it some more. The guidelines I recommend are similar to the American College of Sports Medicine guidelines for strength training for the general population:

- number of sets: 1 to 2
- number of repetitions: 8 to 12
- number of days per week: 1 to 2

I am suggesting you start with one set of 8 to 10 reps for the first two weeks if you have never lifted weights. If you are getting back into it, perform two sets of 8 to 10 reps. If you are already gung ho about weights, start with two sets of 12 reps. Try to get two days of weight training in per week, and I suggest that you do these exercises right after your Kardio. The reason is that you are already in exercise mode, already warmed up (the Kardio counts as your warm-up) and because it is time-efficient. If you choose to weight train on separate days, don't forget the warm-up.

And don't forget to rest. Not only should you ease into weight training, you need to give your muscles 48 hours of rest between workouts. Microscopic tearing occurs in the muscle fibers, which is why you will feel a bit sore sometimes after lifting. Resting allows the muscles to recover and rebuild, which is a part of getting stronger. With this in mind, plan on lifting two days weekly with at least a day in between. If you want to do a shorter weight workout on consecutive days, you could implement workouts called a split routine. A split routine divides the body in two—one day for the upper body and one day for the lower body. Keep in mind that you can do Kardio on back-to-back days, but not weight lifting (unless you are doing split routine).

The Basics

Following is a good basic plan to get you started. Try these exercises for at least one day a week for four weeks, and you should be able to get a good feel for resistance training. A good progression is to work the large muscles first and proceed in descending order. Each of the lower- and upper-body exercises can be executed with dumbbells, although it is a good idea to complete a couple of weeks of lunges and squats without added weight, to prevent undue soreness. And always...

- select an appropriate weight for each exercise

- use proper form when performing an exercise

- use a full range of motion when performing an exercise

- lift and lower the resistance movement in a controlled manner

- hold on to the weights firmly

- breathe rhythmically when performing an exercise, exhaling with the effort and inhaling when returning to the starting point

BASIC WEIGHT-TRAINING PLANS

Lower body:

Lunges (muscles worked—quadriceps, hamstrings, gluteals, and calves)

1. Stand up straight with your feet shoulder-width apart, arms relaxed by your side.

2. Keep your head up (looking ahead) and your abs tight throughout the exercise.

3. Step forward with your right leg and slowly lower your body, while keeping your torso upright.

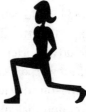

4. Your left foot stays planted while your weight shifts slightly to your toes.

5. Bring your right leg back to the starting position and then do the same movement with your left leg.

Squats (muscles worked—quadriceps, hamstrings, and gluteals)

1. Stand up straight with your feet slightly wider than shoulder-width apart. Point your toes straight ahead or outward, but never inward.

2. Keep your head up (looking ahead) and your abs tight throughout the exercise.

3. Bend your knees and imagine you are sitting down in a chair.

4. Don't drop your hips below your knees and keep your knees from extending over your toes.

5. Stand back up from the squatting position and repeat.

Upper body:

Back—bent-over row (muscles worked—latissimus dorsi, rear deltoids, and biceps)

1. Place your left knee on a bench and your left hand on the same bench in front of you, supporting you in a bent-over position, with your right foot planted on the floor.

2. Your upper torso should be parallel to the floor and the dumbbell near your right foot.

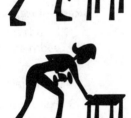

3. Reach down with your right hand and pick up the dumbbell.

4. Imagine you are pulling the handle on an old lawn mower to crank the engine as you pull the dumbbell up to your chest and armpit while keeping your elbow close to your side.

5. Return the dumbbell to its original position and repeat the movement, completing the repetitions.

6. Repeat the same exercise with your left arm as well.

Chest—bench press (muscles worked—pectorals, triceps, and anterior deltoids)

1. Lie flat on your back (you may use the floor or a bench).

2. If necessary, put a towel or pillow behind your neck.

3. Bend your knees and plant your feet firmly on the floor if using a bench.

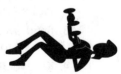

4. Grip the dumbbells (one in each hand) with your hands at chest level and your palms facing your knees.

5. Extend the arms outward without locking the elbows.

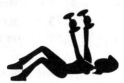

6. Slowly lower the weights back to the chest and repeat.

Shoulders—lateral raise (muscles worked—deltoids)

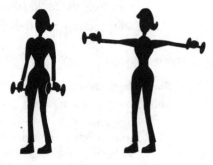

1. Stand up straight with your feet shoulder-width apart.

2. You should have a dumbbell in each hand with your palms facing your outer thighs, arms hanging to the sides.

3. Lift the dumbbells away from your body with your elbows slightly bent until you reach shoulder level.

4. Slowly lower the weights back down to your sides and repeat.

Biceps—biceps curl (muscles worked—biceps)

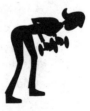

1. Stand up straight with your feet shoulder-width apart, or sit on the edge of a chair.

2. Hold dumbbells in both hands with your palms facing forward.

3. Pull the dumbbells to the top of your shoulders while keeping your elbows at your sides.

4. Slowly lower the weights back to your sides and repeat.

Triceps—triceps kickback (muscles worked—triceps)

1. Stand up straight with your feet shoulder-width apart, or sit on the edge of a chair.

2. Hold dumbbells in both hands with your palms facing your sides.

3. Bend over at the waist with your upper body parallel to the floor.

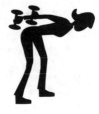

4. Keep your elbows close to your sides and push the dumbbells away from your body (upward).

5. Squeeze the back side of your arms as you complete this movement.

6. Lower the weight back to the starting position and repeat.

Abdominals—abdominal crunches (muscles worked—abdominals, the sheet of muscles on your midsection)

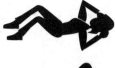

1. Lie flat on the floor on a towel or mat with knees bent and feet flat.
2. Place hands behind head lightly for support.

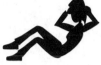

3. Contract your stomach muscles by slowly curling your torso forward, raising your head and shoulder blades off the mat.
4. Hold for one second and lower your upper body back to the starting position and repeat.

Obliques—torso twist (muscles worked—obliques, the external and internal muscles that you use when you rotate the torso from side to side)

1. Start in the same position that you would for a crunch.
2. Instead of curling the torso straight up, twist the torso to the side, rotating one shoulder toward the opposite knee.
3. Think about bringing your elbow to the outside of the opposite knee.

After progressing to two days a week, one set of 12 repetitions of each exercise, add another set of 12 repetitions per muscle group. Don't forget to keep track of the changes in weight lifted as well as sets and reps completed on your weight-training log (see Resources section). Work this program faithfully for four weeks, and then you will be more familiar with your muscles and can safely experiment with other various tools and methods.

Of course, if you love lifting, stick with it, but if you crave developing your muscles with a different discipline, try one of the other options for your second weekly strength training session, like Pilates. Or join one of the many strength-training classes at your local gym or use your body for resistance exercises like pushups. In fact, I use body resistance training for most of my strength-training workouts now because the compound exercises are so time- and place-efficient. See workout below when you are ready to change it up (after four weeks of conventional weight training). My suggestion is to maintain at least one day of this weight training regimen throughout the 12 weeks, with the other strength-training day open for experimentation (such as the option below).

The minimalist body-resistance workout for intermediate to advanced strength level:

1. *Lunges:* 2 sets/12 reps (alternate legs and count until you have repeated 12 reps per leg, take a short rest and repeat)
2. *Pushups:* 2 sets/12 reps
3. *Crunches:* 2 sets/24 reps
4. *Oblique crunches:* 2 sets/24 reps

The intermediate resistance workout for intermediate to advanced strength level:

1. *Lunges:* 2 sets/12 reps
2. *Squats:* 2 sets/12 reps
3. *Pushups:* 2 sets/12 reps
4. *Reverse pushups (a form of dips):* Use a chair, bench, bed, or just the floor to support body weight; bend arms, lower the body, and then return to starting position; 2 sets/12 reps
5. *Crunches:* 1 minute
6. *Oblique crunches:* 1 minute
7. *Reverse crunches:* 1 minute

For those of you still keeping score, "K" is for Kardio, "I" is for intake, "S" is for strength training—and the last "S" could be a book in itself.

"S" Stands for Spirit

Spirit is the cornerstone of the KISS plan. It is the Spirit that gives us the strength, energy, and conviction to do things that we normally could not do. For example, how do we "get gritty" about exercise and eating better amid an already-filled-to-the-brim-and-overflowing cup of activities? Rather than pulling ourselves up by our bootstraps with more self-determination, we start by acknowledging our need and our dependence on God, which reminds me of a verse that I love: " 'Not by might, not by power but by my Spirit' says the LORD." We don't have to embark on this journey of change alone because God is with us and He is for us. "I can do all things *through Him*." The reverse of that is, "*Apart from Him* we can do nothing."[1] You could say either that I'm really convinced of these two verses or I'm really jaded (when it comes to the Spirit). Let me explain what I mean by "jaded."

I am rarely surprised by the bad stuff we can fall into when we are "apart from Him." I've run around the block enough times to see much of the scenery. I'm rarely surprised when relationships unravel because of adultery, sexual promiscuity, or plain selfishness. I'm rarely surprised when justice is not served. Though I'm saddened, I'm usually not surprised by the escalating problem of obesity. These things are tragic, upsetting, and frustrating, but not surprising in light of who we *can* be when we don't rely on God.

Watch how this plays out on the flip side. I'm not often stunned by the amazing things that happen "through Him." In other words, when marriages that are founded in religion work, I'm thrilled, but not stunned. I sort of expect people who have given their lives over to God to change for the better. I'm not surprised when families or friends are reunited, emotions and addictions are healed, or when people change the way they eat and exercise. These things are so exciting, moving, and encouraging, but not shocking in light of who we *can* be. That's who we can be when the Spirit is working in us and through us.

Apart from Him we can do nothing, but *through Him* we can do all things, especially change for the better. In this case by surrendering ourselves and our lifestyles to God, we can "make exercise and eating well happen."

I think it's important to mention two of the many things about "through Him" that we can apply to our weight-loss goals. First, *"through Him" begins with prayer,* and praying for God's help is an essential element of change.

Here's a simple starting point:

> Dear God,
>
> I acknowledge that You are God and You are in control of everything. I need Your strength and Your power to overcome my battle with food and weight loss. I confess that I am weak and that You are strong. Empower me to eat, drink, and exercise in a way that honors You.
>
> In Jesus' name, amen.

Second, *"through Him" is also carried out in community.* Life is lived in community, and we could catch an exercise and eating clue from this. One of the most neglected components of weight loss and keeping fit is community. We Americans value rugged individualism—"I am the diva of my own story." No doubt you have to take personal responsibility for your weight loss, but equally important is enlisting the help of others for mutual accountability.

There are many ways you can exercise in community. To name a few:

- Get a partner to run, walk, or lift weights with.
- Join a Pilates or spinning class.
- Find some friends and start your own workout group, such as Boot Camp.
- Hire a personal trainer, if your budget allows.

Exercising in community will create accountability for you. It's much easier for me to skip an 8 AM workout if I am doing it on my own, but if I have a partner who is expecting to meet me, I will be much more likely to get my bed-head self there. Plus, we all need encouragement along the way to make our goals. Let's face it, life often beats us down, and when that happens many times we turn to food and away from exercising. Having a group of friends or at a least a partner, will help get you back on track when you fall off the workout wagon. God didn't design us to live life and face its challenges alone. The communal God designed us to live in a replenishing community.

You Can Change!

The good news is that by the grace of God and with His strength you can change. I certainly have. The fact that eating nutritiously is second nature to me now is a radical departure from my old diet of junk food and Diet Coke. From exercising only when I "felt" like it to exercising consistently, I've changed. I'm not saying I have arrived or that I am immune to setbacks and temptations. I haven't reached my destination, but I am certainly not where I started. I'm not where I want to be, but I'm not where I was! It's like any important area of life—there will always be a tension to "keep it real."

Take marriage, for example. You can be on cloud 999 one moment, awed by how harmoniously one you are with your "soul mate," and thinking, *I've got the marriage thing down—what's so hard about it?* The next thing you know, out of nowhere, it starts unraveling. You're thinking, *You're not the man/woman I thought you were.* Your communication is off, your priorities aren't in sync, your partner is not meeting your needs, and you are not "feeling the love." Suddenly, marriage is hard. What do you do? Do you throw in the towel, or do you ask for God's help, "commit to grit," and get to work?

Another comparison could be our spiritual journey. When we have an "experience" with Christ, we usually have a honeymoon phase where all of our prayers seem to be answered, the spiritual "highs" far outweigh any lows, the victories outnumber the defeats, every day is an exciting opportunity to "live for God" and to "rejoice in the Lord." Life is good...until one day trials begin to come your way. Like Job, who lost all his cattle and his children in a day, we feel the Lord has abandoned us. Or is He just "keeping it real"? My take on the phrase "keeping it real" involves embracing the tensions of every good thing, every gift, every joy, and every blessing, knowing they can all change with the tide. That's why our faith must be grounded, not in things, but in the person of Christ. *That's* keeping it real—because He never changes, and He is with us always. Think about this every day of your weight-loss journey:

> **"Your worst days are never so bad that you are beyond the reach of God's grace. And your best days are never so good that you are beyond the need of God's grace."**
>
> *—Jerry Bridges*

I have prayed for those of you reading this story. Whatever you do, don't get back on the dieting treadmill—as you know it will take you nowhere. It's high time to kiss dieting goodbye and embrace the new you…the new you fully committed to the new way to KISS!

WILL'S STORY

My husband and I love to hear success stories from people who have kissed dieting goodbye, shed the pounds, and kept them off.

Will struggled with weight issues for more than ten years. He grew up in a divided home. Not only were his parents divorced, but his mom was thin and his dad was obese. When he attended graduate school, he gained 35 pounds. But it was not till he started his career as an accountant that he began to notice the pattern. After a stressful day of work or a tension-filled meeting he would head straight for the vending machine or the closest convenience store and binge on candy bars and doughnuts. This continued until he was in his mid-30s, when he realized he had to do something about his weight and crazy eating habits.

So, like most of us, he jumped on the diet roller coaster. Losing pounds and gaining them back—the thrill of victory and the agony of defeat—became his way of life. Finally, he realized the problem wasn't grounded in his stomach or in food, but in his mind. As he says, "I came to realize that the word *diet* truly is a four-letter word. Dieting is *not* the solution for someone who's overweight."

After his enlightenment, Will kissed dieting goodbye and made a lifelong commitment to embracing the disciplines of exercise and nutritious food. He developed a simple but effective approach to losing weight and keeping it off:

- He got in touch with the emotional triggers that caused him to overeat.

- He jumped on the treadmill or went for a swim after stressful events, and he even planned his Kardio session around potential triggers.

- He made better choices about food and kept healthy snacks handy.

- He kept a journal of his workouts, food intake, and emotions surrounding the day's events.

- He started eating five to six small meals a day, which kept the cravings at bay and also stabilized his blood sugar.

A couple of years ago, Will had a setback, and his good habits went packing. Inevitably, he packed on the pounds again. Instead of throwing in the towel, though, he got back into his Kardio habit, altered his eating to fit the needs of his body, and got to losing again. Today, I'm proud to report that he's keeping the pounds off and training for a marathon.

Will has learned how to make it happen.

I want to encourage you on your journey. Don't give up the fight against flab. Don't let rough seasons keep you from KISSing. You can do it. You now have the tools to lose excess weight, eat healthily, and get into shape in a way that impacts every area of your life for the better. You will feel better, look better, and live better. I am cheering for you and praying for victory. So now...*make it happen!*

Resources for KISSing

Body Mass Index

The body mass index (BMI) classifies appropriate weight and levels of overweight. A BMI of 19 to 24.9 indicates that you are at a healthy weight. If your BMI is between 25 and 29.9 you are considered overweight, and a BMI of 30 or higher is indicative of obesity.

The chart on page 209 helps you find your BMI.[1] Look for your height in the left-hand column. Scan to the right to find your weight in order to determine whether or not you fall into the appropriate range. The number at the top of the chart is your BMI.

Weight (lb.)

BMI	19	20	21	22	23	24	25	26	27	28	29	30	31	32	33	34	35	36	37	38	39
Height (in.)																					
58	91	96	100	105	110	115	119	124	129	134	138	143	148	153	158	162	167	172	177	181	186
59	94	99	104	109	114	119	124	128	133	138	143	148	153	158	163	168	173	178	183	188	193
60	97	102	107	112	118	123	128	133	138	143	148	153	158	163	168	174	179	184	189	194	199
61	100	106	111	116	122	127	132	137	143	148	153	158	164	169	174	180	185	190	195	201	206
62	104	109	115	120	126	131	136	142	147	153	158	164	169	175	180	186	191	196	202	207	213
63	107	113	118	124	130	135	141	146	152	158	163	169	175	180	186	191	197	203	208	214	220
64	110	116	122	128	134	140	145	151	157	163	169	174	180	186	192	197	204	209	215	221	227
65	114	120	126	132	138	144	150	156	162	168	174	180	186	192	198	204	210	216	222	228	234
66	118	124	130	136	142	148	155	161	167	173	179	186	192	198	204	210	216	223	229	235	241
67	121	127	134	140	146	153	159	166	172	178	185	191	198	204	211	217	223	230	236	242	249
68	125	131	138	144	151	158	164	171	177	184	190	197	203	210	216	223	230	236	243	249	256
69	128	135	142	149	155	162	169	176	182	189	196	203	209	216	223	230	236	243	250	257	263
70	132	139	146	153	160	167	174	181	188	195	202	209	216	222	229	236	243	250	257	264	271
71	136	143	150	157	165	172	179	186	193	200	208	215	222	229	236	243	250	257	265	272	279
72	140	147	154	162	169	177	184	191	199	206	213	221	228	235	242	250	258	265	272	279	287
73	144	151	159	166	174	182	189	197	204	212	219	227	234	242	250	257	265	272	280	288	295
74	148	155	163	171	179	186	194	202	210	218	225	233	241	249	256	264	272	280	287	295	303
75	152	160	168	176	184	192	200	208	216	224	232	240	248	256	264	272	279	287	295	303	311
76	156	164	172	180	189	197	205	213	221	230	238	246	254	263	271	279	287	295	304	312	320

Goal-Setting Chart

First, see *SAM* at the beginning of chapter 12 in regard to setting goals.*

Starting weight: _____

Weight-loss goal for the month: _____

Long-term weight-loss goal (12 weeks): _____

Week 1   Weight at the beginning of the week: _____
Weight-loss goal for the week: _____
Eating goal for the week:
Exercise goal for the week:

Week 2   Weight at the beginning of the week: _____
Weight-loss goal for the week: _____
Eating goal for the week:
Exercise goal for the week:

Week 3   Weight at the beginning of the week: _____
Weight-loss goal for the week: _____
Eating goal for the week:
Exercise goal for the week:

Week 4   Weight at the beginning of the week: _____
Weight-loss goal for the week: _____
Eating goal for the week:
Exercise goal for the week:

Week 5   Weight at the beginning of the week: _____
Weight-loss goal for the week: _____
Eating goal for the week:
Exercise goal for the week:

Week 6   Weight at the beginning of the week: _____

Weight-loss goal for the week: _____

Eating goal for the week:

Exercise goal for the week:

Week 7   Weight at the beginning of the week: _____

Weight-loss goal for the week: _____

Eating goal for the week:

Exercise goal for the week:

Week 8   Weight at the beginning of the week: _____

Weight-loss goal for the week: _____

Eating goal for the week:

Exercise goal for the week:

Week 9   Weight at the beginning of the week: _____

Weight-loss goal for the week: _____

Eating goal for the week:

Exercise goal for the week:

Week 10   Weight at the beginning of the week: _____

Weight-loss goal for the week: _____

Eating goal for the week:

Exercise goal for the week:

Week 11   Weight at the beginning of the week: _____

Weight-loss goal for the week: _____

Eating goal for the week:

Exercise goal for the week:

Week 12   Weight at the beginning of the week: _____

Weight-loss goal for the week: _____

Eating goal for the week:

Exercise goal for the week:

Exercise Journal:
Kardio

Write down the mode of exercise (Stairmaster, treadmill, and so on), record your heart rate, the amount of time spent exercising, and how you felt after exercise. The following is a one-week sample.*

	Mode of exercise	Intensity (THR)	Time	How I felt afterward
Week 1 _____ to _____ (date) (date)				
Sunday _____ (date)				
Monday _____ (date)				
Tuesday _____ (date)				
Wednesday _____ (date)				
Thursday _____ (date)				
Friday _____ (date)				
Saturday _____ (date)				

Exercise Journal:
Weight Training

Write down the muscle worked, the specific exercise performed, the amount of weight, and the sets and repetitions completed. Commit to journaling your workouts for 12 weeks. The following is a one-week sample.*

	Muscle group	Exercise	Weight	Sets/Reps
Week 1 _____ to _____ (date) (date)				
Sunday _____ (date)				
Monday _____ (date)				
Tuesday _____ (date)				
Wednesday _____ (date)				
Thursday _____ (date)				
Friday _____ (date)				
Saturday _____ (date)				

Food Journal

List only the fruits, vegetables, and Super Foods consumed per meal to see how well you are feeding your body.*

Week 1

_____ to _____
(date)   (date)

Sunday _____
          (date)

breakfast

lunch

dinner

Monday _____
          (date)

breakfast

lunch

dinner

Tuesday _____
          (date)

breakfast

lunch

dinner

---

* Permission to copy this chart for personal use only is granted to the purchaser of this book.

Wednesday _____
              (date)

breakfast

lunch

dinner

Thursday _____
              (date)

breakfast

lunch

dinner

Friday _____
              (date)

breakfast

lunch

dinner

Saturday _____
              (date)

breakfast

lunch

dinner

Super Foods List

Remember that Super Foods, compared to other foods, have a high nutrient density for the amount of calories they contain. In other words, they are nutrition-packed and can help you feel good and lose weight.

Here are some of the popular Super Foods, though this list is not exhaustive:

yogurt

tea (green or black)

flaxseed

broccoli

beans

tomatoes

walnuts

oats

soy

quinoa

salmon

spinach

blueberries

grapefruit

pomegranates

sweet potatoes

oranges

pumpkin

lentils

turkey

apples

avocados

kiwi fruit

olives and extra-virgin olive oil

tuna

trout

whole grains

concord grapes

cranberries

omega-3 eggs

watermelon

NOTES

Chapter 1—Kiss Failure Goodbye

1. Amanda Spake, "Stop Dieting!" *U.S. News and World Report,* January 16, 2006.
2. Peter Doskoch, "The Winning Edge," *Psychology Today* magazine, Nov./Dec. 2005.

Chapter 2—Kiss Craziness Goodbye

1. Margaret Shannon, *Gullible's Troubles* (Boston: Houghton Mifflin Co., 1998).
2. Barbara Kantrowitz and Claudia Kalb, "Food News Blues," *Newsweek,* March 13, 2006, pp. 44, 55.
3. Gina Kolata, "Low-Fat Diet Does Not Cut Health Risks, Study Finds," *New York Times,* February 8, 2006.
4. H. Leighton Steward, Morrison C. Bethea, M.D., Sam S. Andrews, M.D., Luis A. Balart, M.D., *Sugar Busters!: Cut Sugar to Trim Fat* (New York: Random House, 1998), p. 13.
5. Genesis 1:29 NIV.
6. See Genesis 9:3-4 NIV.

Chapter 3—Kiss I*diet*ry Goodbye

Epigraph: Isaiah 43:18 NIV.
1. Genesis 2:9 NIV.
2. Romans 7:15.
3. Romans 7:4-6.
4. Colossians 2:21-23.
5. 1 Peter 4:1-2.
6. See 1 Peter 5:5.
7. See James 2:13.
8. 1 Corinthians 15:32.
9. Proverbs 3:5-6.

Chapter 4—Kiss Perfection Goodbye

Epigraph: Psalm 139:13-15.

1. Boston Women's Health Collective, *Our Bodies, Our Selves* (New York: Simon & Schuster, 2005), p. 7.
2. Boston Women's Health Collective.
3. Susan Block, "Starving in Silence," *American School Board Journal,* March 2002.
4. Genesis 3:6.
5. C.S. Lewis, *The Screwtape Letters* (San Francisco: Harper San Francisco, 2001), p. 20.
6. See 1 Samuel 16:7.
7. Leslie Goldman, "Special Report on Weight and Body Image," *Weight Watchers,* May/June 2006, p. 113.
8. Goldman.
9. Boston Women's Health Collective, p. 7.
10. Goldman.
11. Boston Women's Health Collective, p. 10.
12. See John 8:32.
13. John 1:14.
14. Wayne Grudem, *Bible Doctrine* (Grand Rapids, MI: Zondervan), p. 262.
15. See John 14:16,26.
16. Romans 12:1 NASB.
17. 2 Corinthians 4:7.

Chapter 5—Kiss the Couch Goodbye

1. Arthur Blessit, "How Far Did Jesus and Mary Walk?" www.blessitt.com/jesuswalked.html, March 15, 2006.
2. "Nutrition Action Healthletter," *Journal of Applied Physiology,* December 2005.
3. Melvin H. Williams, *Nutrition for Fitness and Sport: Fourth Edition,* ed. Edward Bartell (Dubuque, IA: Brown and Benchmark), p. 318.
4. Judith A. DeCava, "Getting Physical," *Nutrition News and Views,* March/April 2000, p. 1.

Chapter 6—Kiss Flab Goodbye

Epigraph: Proverbs 31:17, 25 NIV.

1. Proverbs 31:17 AMP.
2. Judith A. DeCava, "Getting Physical," *Nutrition News and Views,* March/April 2000, p. 6.
3. DeCava, p. 4.
4. 2 Corinthians 4:16.
5. Ralph Pafferbarger Jr., *Nutrition News,* as quoted in DeCava, p. 3.

Chapter 7—Embrace Random Acts

Epigraph: 1 Corinthians 9:22 NASB 1977.

1. 1 Corinthians 9:27.
2. *Journal of the American Medical Association,* vol. 289 (2003): p. 1795; as quoted in Bonnie Liebmann, "While You Wait: The Cost of Inactivity," *Nutrition Action Health Letter,* December 2005, p. 6; Melvin H. Williams, *Nutrition for Fitness and Sport: Fourth Edition,* ed. Edward Bartell (Dubuque, IA: Brown and Benchmark), p. 318.
3. Taken from Associated Press, "Obese Man Ends Cross-Country Health Trek," www.msnbc.msn.com/id/127li006/, posted on May 10, 2006.
4. Adapted from guidelines developed by the American College of Sports Medicine.

Chapter 8—Embrace Food

1. Ephesians 5:29.
2. Romans 12:1 NASB; 1 Corinthians 6:19-20.
3. Genesis 1:29,31.
4. Psalm 104:14-16.
5. See, respectively, Matthew 4:4; 1 Kings 17:15-16; Luke 9:16; Matthew 26:26; Luke 24:30; 1 Corinthians 10.
6. See, respectively, Exodus 24:11; Genesis 31:54; Genesis 41; John 2.
7. See Matthew 26:26; 1 Corinthians 11:24.
8. Deuteronomy 8:7-18.
9. See Genesis 18.
10. Adapted from Miriam Feinberg Vamosh, *Food at the Times of Bible: From Adam's Apple to The Last Supper* (Herzlia, Israel: Phalpot Ltd. and Abingdon Press, 2004), p. 94.

Chapter 9—Embrace Nutritious

1. *Nutrition News and Views,* January 2006, p. 2.
2. Rodale Women's Health Group, "Lose Weight Now," *Prevention,* 2005, p. 17.
3. Rodale Women's Health Group, pp. 4-5.
4. *American Journal of Clinical Nutrition,* 1 January 2005, pp. 122-129.
5. Taken from the Supplement Chart in Michael Murray, Joseph Pizzorno, Lara Pizzorno, *The Encyclopedia of Healing Foods* (New York: Atria, 2005), p. 749.
6. Rodale Women's Health Group, p. 12.
7. Murray, Pizzorno, Pizzorno, pp. 328-329.
8. *Journal of the American College of Nutrition,* 2005, vol. 24, no. 3.
9. Taken from www.holisticonline.com/Remedies/weight/weight_common-sense-recommendations.htm, June 1, 2006.
10. Murray, Pizzorno, Pizzorno, *Healing Foods,* p. 231.
11. Murray, Pizzorno, Pizzorno, *Healing Foods,* pp. 259-260.
12. Jane Clarke, "At Your Table: Pomegranates," *London Times,* September 24, 2005.

Chapter 10—Embrace Fresh

1. Ronald L. Prior, USDA Agriculture Research Service, as quoted in *Prevention* magazine, February 2006, p. 73.
2. "When it pays to buy organic," *Consumer Reports on Health,* February 2006.
3. *Journal of Agricultural and Food Chemistry,* February 26, 2003, as found on www.mercola.com.

Chapter 11—Embrace Satisfaction

Epigraph: Excerpted from the song "You Created." © Joshua Moore. Used by permission. All rights reserved.

1. John Rosemond, *Six-Point Plan for Raising Happy, Healthy Children* (Kansas City: Andrews and McMeel, 1989), pp. 67,68.
2. Eric Schlosser, *Fast Food Nation* (New York: Harper Perennial), pp. 56,57.
3. Taken from Tod Barrett, "House Bans Fast-Food Lawsuits," CNN Washington Bureau, as found on www.supersizeme.com.
4. Judith A. DeCava, "Food, Youth, and Truth," *Nutrition News and Views,* May/June 2003, p. 1.
5. DeCava, p. 1.
6. Titus 1:12; Philippians 3:19.
7. Isaiah 55:1-2 NASB.
8. Psalm 23:1.
9. "Why You Can't Eat Just One," *Consumer Reports on Health,* March 2006, p. 10.
10. C.S. Lewis, *The Lion, the Witch, and the Wardrobe* (New York: Harper Collins, 1978), pp. 38, 39.
11. Galatians 5:22-23.
12. Taken from B. Barkeling, Y. Linne, E. Melin, and P. Rooth, "Vision and Eating Behavior in Obese Subjects," *Obesity,* January 1, 2003, pp. 130-134.
13. "The New American Plate: Standard Serving Size Finder," www.aicr.org.
14. Mary Dwenwald, "Imagine Never Having to Go on Another Diet for the Rest of Your Life, Ever Again," *Real Simple,* February 2005, p. 162.

Chapter 12—The New Way to KISS

1. Zechariah 4:6; Philippians 4:13 NASB; paraphrase of John 15:5.

Resources for KISSing

1. Adapted from National Heart, Lung, and Blood Institute, *Clinical Guidelines on the Identification, Evaluation, and Treatment of Overweight and Obesity in Adults* (NIH Publication No. 98-4083).

About the Author

Elliott Young is a personal trainer certified by the Cooper Institute, with a master's degree in exercise and health-related fitness. Her own battle with destructive dieting cycles eventually led her to discover a healthy and holistic alternative. She is also a speaker and mentor, and lives in Texas with her husband, Ben, and their two daughters.

For more information, or to book Elliott for a speaking engagement, contact:

Toni Richmond
Second Baptist Church
6400 Woodway
Houston, TX 77057
713.465.3408

Information is also available at Elliott's Web site:

www.kissdietinggoodbye.com

Want to gain energy, lose weight, and enjoy better health?

For author Dennis Pollock, the idea of losing both of his legs to diabetes—like his mother had—wasn't a pleasant prospect. But after experiencing his own frightening symptoms of out-of-control blood sugar, he had to make a choice: get control of his diet and exercise, or pay the price down the road.

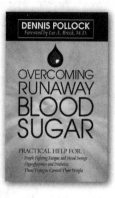

Thankfully, Dennis has found a successful answer for blood-sugar fluctuations. With his positive, can-do approach, you too can gain maximum health while losing excess pounds. You'll discover...

- why runaway blood sugar is a key factor in food cravings and weight issues
- how blood-sugar problems lead to damage to your body
- ways to evaluate pre-diabetes health risks, such as hypoglycemia
- reasons and motivation to change your lifestyle
- diet and exercise that really work

Whether you are diabetic, have a family history of diabetes, or are simply tired of being sick and tired, *Overcoming Runaway Blood Sugar* may very well change the way you view eating and exercise forever.

> *"Dennis Pollock is offering practical advice*
> *to help you move toward healthy living."*
> —from the foreword by Lee A. Brock, MD

A changed life begins with small changes

Are you trying to discover a healthier, more balanced life? In *7 Simple Steps to a Healthier You,* Dawn Hall, creator of the popular Busy People's Cookbooks series (more than 1 million copies sold) offers a new way of thinking, eating, and moving that can turn today's motivation into lasting health and wholeness. Dawn shows you how to

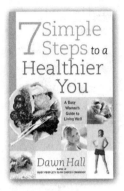

- identify and make the simple choices that lead to success
- design a 7-step personal plan that ensures commitment and results
- create healthy meals with easy recipes and fabulous tips

Whether this encouraging and realistic approach is used as a complete program or as a complement to your own regimen, a healthier *you* is just steps away.

Renew your mind Rejuvenate your body

Would you like to increase your flexibility, improve your circulation, and enhance your level of energy? Finally there's a program that offers proven streching and flexibility exercises without troubling Eastern influences. Now you can fill your mind with the Word of God as you practice the postures on this DVD that will

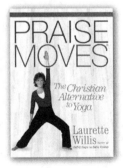

- promote healing and overall physical health
- relieve stress and enhance relaxation
- glorify God with your spirit, soul, and body

Certified personal trainer Laurette Willis shows you a way to transform your workouts into worship with *PraiseMoves*™!

When food starts to control your life

Food and sex, as well as other good things created by God, can be misused in order to run away from emotional/relational pain. When this happens, the resulting damage, desperation, and loneliness can be worse than the worst nightmare...for you or someone you care about.

Using groundbreaking research and offering compassionate understanding rooted deeply in the Bible, David Eckman shares

Sex Food & God

Breaking Free from Temptations, Compulsions, & Addictions

David Eckman

- how and why unhealthy appetites grip and trap people in a fantasy world
- how shame and guilt disappear when we realize how much God delights in us
- how four great experiences of the spiritual life break the addiction cycle

As you begin to grasp God's radical plan for freedom, you'll find yourself wanting to run *toward* Him—and away from aloneness and self-deception.

"David Eckman is a man you can trust...His teaching resonates with God's wisdom and compassion."

—Stu Weber, author of *Tender Warrior*